LUCK IS NO LONGER MY SHADOW

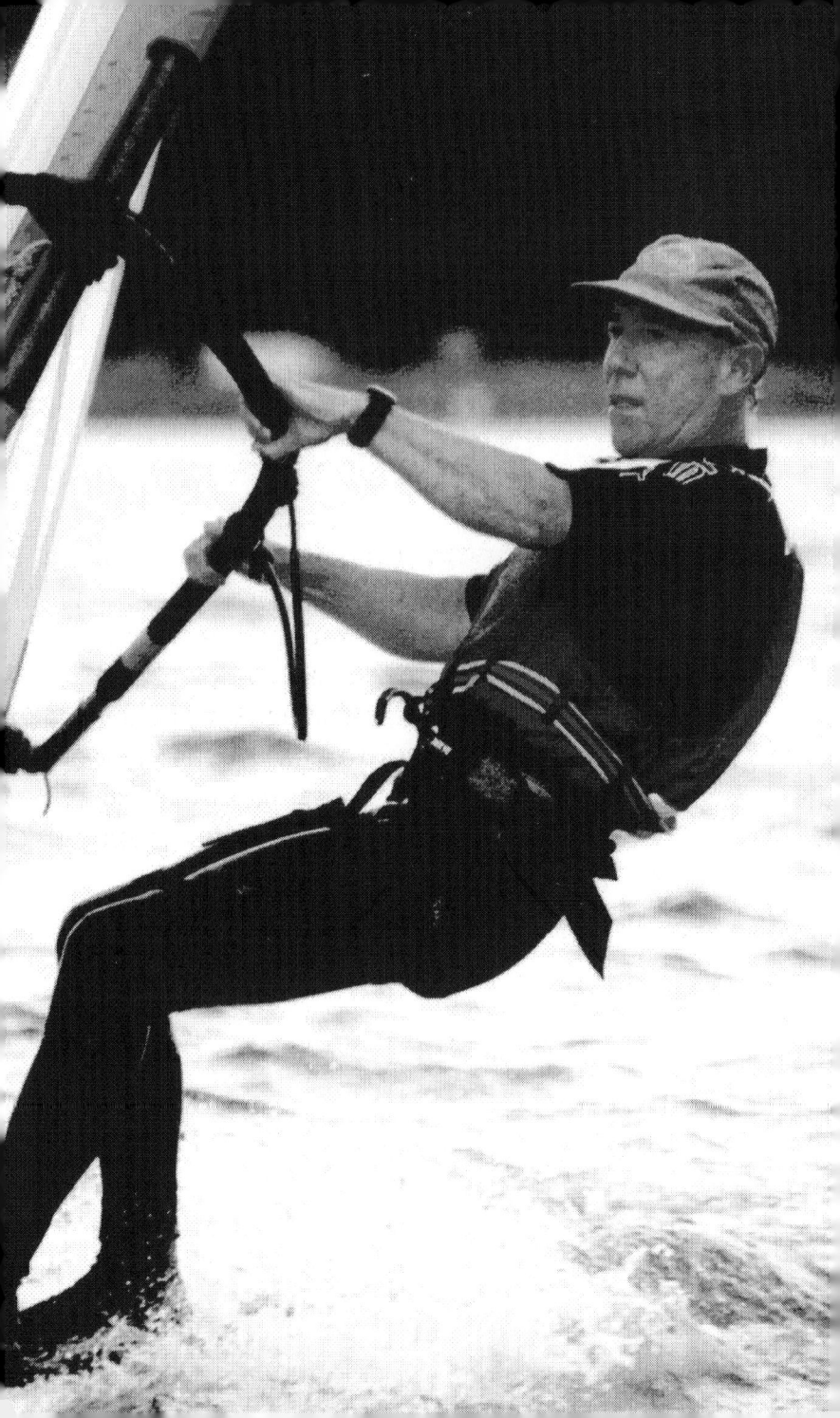

About the Author

Terry Adcock became a pilot at the age of seventeen and joined the Royal Air Force. At the age of twenty he became a bomber captain with a nuclear role. Later he became an instructor, a display pilot, and Wing Commander, commanding two fighter squadrons. Uniquely for a member of the RAF, he sailed across the world as a member of a sea-going Admiral's staff. The story of this active career is told in his book "Luck is my Shadow".

After his career in the RAF he managed airborne-weapons research and European and UK airspace projects.

What People Thought of "Luck Is No Longer My Shadow"

"This book made me both laugh and cry. It is about love (real love). It tells of a life led by principle, passion and perseverance: passion for flying and his sport; love for his family; dogged determination to keep his family alive and safe when the rules governing key institutions mitigated against him; and the struggle to keep fit so that he could accomplish all else.

Not only does the tale between the covers give warning to people caring for ailing relatives of difficulties that might lie ahead, but it may also inspire people beginning retirement to do something worthwhile with their remaining years: whether it be to take up a new sport or hobby, to embark on a new career, or even to write a book or invent a useful gadget. All of these Terry Adcock did.

I hope you enjoy the book as much as I did."

Maya Chatterjee
(retired school teacher)

"Moving, poignant and relevant in equal measure"

Malcolm V. Angel
(owner of Gulliver's Book Store in Wimborne Minster, Dorset)

"I found the book extremely interesting and very readable. I could well relate to the problems Terry had with the NHS. I suppose it would be heartless of me to say I enjoyed the book, but it certainly held my attention to the very last page; I really found it difficult to put down when I needed to do other things."

Pauline Dixon
(retired civil servant)

"This is a story about a life led to the full with all its ups and downs. Some of the later chapters about the care home and the treatment of his first wife were quite hard to read."

Pamela Kinnear
(retired primary school teacher)

"By the end of the book, the title's meaning became very clear, but Terry spent many years in retirement fighting it."

Patricia Pitts
(retired magistrate)

Copyright © 2024 by Terry Adcock

All rights reserved. No part of this book may be reproduced or used in any manner without written permission of the copyright owner except for the use of quotations in a book review. For more information, contact:
publishing@publishingpush.com

First paperback edition 2024

978-1-80541-572-5 – eBook
978-1-80541-573-2 – hardcover
978-1-80541-574-9 - paperback

LUCK IS NO LONGER MY SHADOW

When Life Must Change From
One of Duty to a Duty of Care

Terry Adcock

Acknowledgements

Mary and I met in old age, and we thought we would be lucky to survive together for a few years, but we survived against the difficult odds of Parkinson's, deafness and cancer, to name just a few hurdles. Loneliness was pushed back and out of sight.

My thanks also to my family, who have tolerated my idiosyncrasies, and to my many friends who have made me laugh away the difficult times over a cup of coffee.

Many thanks to The Leonardo Trust, a local organisation in Dorset providing support to the county's carers. Understanding and sympathy were given to me when the weight of caring, age and serious health problems were at a high level.

Finally, my thanks to Maya Chatterjee, who strongly believed that my journal should be read by a wide audience and enabled this book to be published.

My general message: the second half of life is so different from the first.

Man plans and God laughs

"No matter what is planned in the middle years for retirement and old age, things will almost certainly turn out to be quite different."

Terry's Family Tree (abridged)

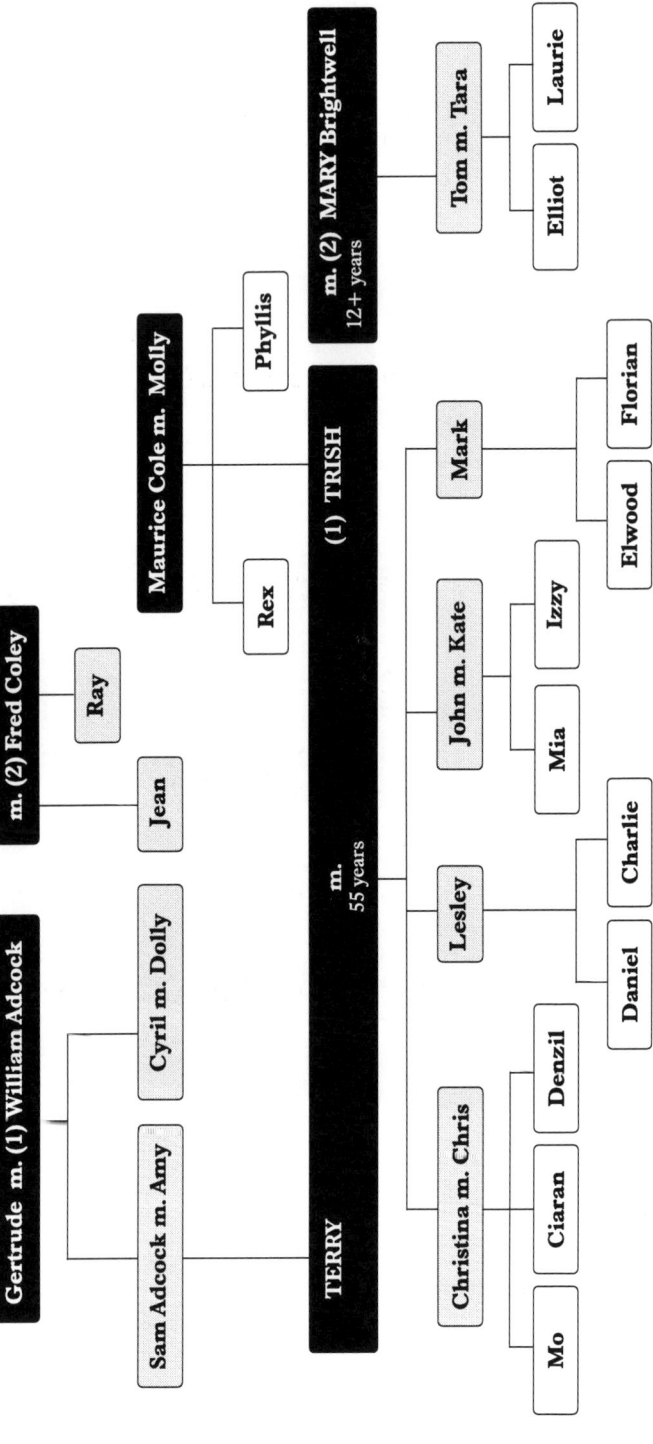

Contents

Prologue — 1
The Transition

Chapter One — 5
Houses, New Jobs and Schools

Chapter Two — 15
Windsurfing

Chapter Three — 45
Hatfield, Computers and the SDI

Chapter Four — 55
Stevenage and a Recession

Chapter Five — 59
The National Air Traffic Service

Chapter Six — 67
The Start of Our Travels

Chapter Seven — 75
Retirement to Dorset and Dramatic Changes

Chapter Eight — 89
The Future and a Glance Back

Chapter Nine — 93
Parkinson's

Chapter Ten — 99
Caring and Old Age

Chapter Eleven — 105
A Horrible Decision

Chapter Twelve — 107
The NHS Has Problems

Chapter Thirteen — 113
Trish Goes Into a Home

Chapter Fourteen — 117
Care and Finance

Chapter Fifteen — 121
Care Becomes Dangerous

Chapter Sixteen — 125
A Doctor Makes Me Very Angry

Chapter Seventeen — 131
I Treat Dropped Head Syndrome

Chapter Eighteen — 135
I Decide to Sell the Family House

Chapter Nineteen — 143
Christmas 2012

Chapter Twenty — 147
Professional Support Is Awful

Chapter Twenty-One — 153
Trish Dies

Chapter Twenty-Two — 155
The Lady Upstairs

Chapter Twenty-Three **Married Again: a Five-Year Contract**	**163**
Chapter Twenty-Four **My Cardiac Sky**	**167**
Chapter Twenty-Five **Old Age and Health Issues**	**171**
Chapter Twenty-Six **The Pandemic**	**177**
Chapter Twenty-Seven **The World Is Broken, the UK Is Broken, the NHS Is Broken; We Fight On**	191
Epilogue **Accepting the Inevitable**	197
Abbreviations Used	199
Glossary	201
Additional Information	201

Prologue
The Transition

The first forty-seven years of my life were packed with excitement, as recorded in my book *Luck Is My Shadow* published in 2020. The interesting part of that life, which was somewhat similar to that of a footballer or athlete, was the problem of getting older, and I had to adapt. True, I could have stayed on and served my time in the MOD as a policymaker or something similar, but it wasn't really me and there were also other aspects of life that were becoming increasingly important. I had learnt a lesson about my dedication to work which, if continued, would break my marriage. Then there was the way the armed forces were dwindling, and my disagreement about the production of the next generation of fighter aircraft. I thought there would always be international upheaval and we were not taking the right road with defence. Of course, I was not alone in my views, and I was supported into a civilian job that was to allow me to pursue my ideas.

On my dining-out night from the RAF, at the Horse Guards Hotel, I was to give a speech that caused the staffs to go back to the MOD and investigate my thoughts about the way things were looking.

After making my case, I excused myself by saying I had a train to catch to a new life. It was an arrogant statement about leaving the RAF, but it chimed with the great confidence I had about the future. I strode down the stairs from the fifth floor of the MOD main building and, for a few moments, just stood at the top of the steps at the entrance drinking in cool air and feeling pleased with myself. I should have noticed there were dark clouds in the distance and suddenly there was a flash of lightning, followed by the rumble of thunder and the rain fell. I shrugged and strode off to King's Cross. I did not wish to consider the portent of dark clouds on the horizon. They just did not exist.

Initially, I thought little about this incident, but over the years I have given it much more thought. Perhaps nature had given me a salutary reminder that no one has any idea about the future, but I had ignored the weather warning received on those steps.

When I was twenty years old, I thought it was difficult to find a life after thirty because my friends had died so early, but here I was aged forty-seven striding out to another life. As this book shows, life was to change quite dramatically.

In the past, I had gone out of my way to seek excitement and risk in the air and at sea. I loved every minute of it, even though I had come close to leaving this world a few times. But the big change came.

Everything was to be different. True, for a few years, I continued to take risks and look for excitement, but then I had to stop looking for physical risk and being selfish. Slowly, the risk and excitement disappeared. I grew up and had to think about taking care of others and encountered a very different problem and another form of survival.

Chapter One
Houses, New Jobs and Schools

In 1983, while I was still in the RAF, Trish (my first wife) and I decided we should get into the property market. For the first time, we bought a family home: a five-bedroom cottage (the Old Post Office) in Market Rasen. We had picked that village as a starting point because it was not far from RAF Binbrook on the Lincolnshire Wolds, where I had completed my last flying tour. It enabled an easy first move and the boys' prep school was close by. Initially, I gritted my teeth when commuting to the MOD in London and, in many ways, it hastened my decision to leave the RAF.

I put up with commuting for a few months but eventually moved into a flat overlooking Buckingham Palace Mews with other MOD desk officers. It was an extremely hard-working time in many ways, because the cottage was in bad repair and the weekends were spent rectifying walls and ceilings that were unsafe. Also, there was an acre of land with a very large, dilapidated greenhouse and vines. We built a garage too. In the background was my work in the MOD: writing a case to prevent yet another reduction in manpower;

the long-term plans for the RAF in the backwash of the Falklands War; and the selection of the first British person to head into space. It was heady stuff.

In August 1984 I stepped out into my new civilian life. In some ways it was like a posting, which had been a way of life in the past. We worked to sell and move to achieve more stability. However, during the first few months of our new life an unwanted letter arrived addressed to Trish. I knew who had sent it; there were tears and it was a no-looking-back watershed. As a result, Trish fell into my arms, and we became totally committed to the family again. It was a close-run thing. Trish and I worked together to make things happen to meet family needs. The boys were on summer holiday as we started the change, and their new term would be at Bedford School.[1] There was no messing about. Our first house at Osgodby was soon sold, as was Mum's house in Norfolk, and the finances were combined with a commuted pension and small mortgage, enabling us to look for another house within bus distance of Bedford School.

My mother was to join us. That sent Trish to look

---

1 Trish was very keen on state education and we both would have liked to have the boys follow us and settle into a grammar school, but we could not envisage that as a possibility. The girls had suffered from my RAF career, and we wanted stability above all else. It was a hard-learnt lesson. It was also a bit late for a family home because the girls were already in their twenties.

for a teaching job, which she found at Sandy en route to the boys' school.

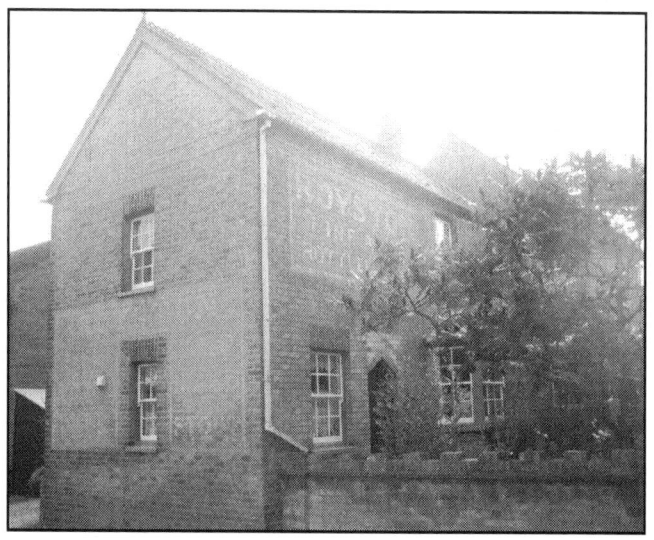

Our second house (in Gamlingay), a seventeenth-century alehouse called "The Three Horseshoes"

We a found a house in Gamlingay, a small peaceful country village.[2] The house was an old seventeenth century alehouse called The 3 Horseshoes. I guess locals visited to have their jugs filled.

---

2   Gamlingay has the honour of an entry in the Guinness Book of Records for being the most misspelt village in the UK. It also has one of the best documented histories over a 1000-year existence. Much of the village has been, and is still, owned by Merton College, Oxford.

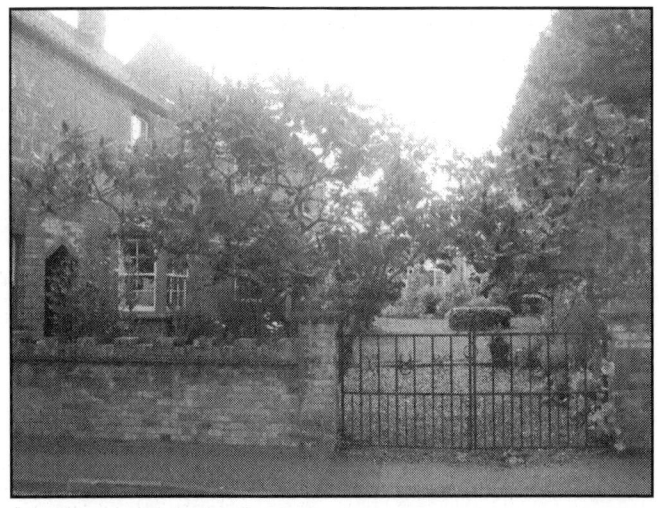

The house in Gamlingay

We all fell in love with it because it had something for all the members of the family. The boys had their own rooms, which they chose without argument, and we agreed they could decorate them, within certain rules, how they wanted. There was also a cellar that was soon eyed up for their projects and a room for the girls to visit. Outside there was an ample garden with a well and an orchard Trish could call her own, and garages and sheds that revived dormant feelings in me for boat-building, but they were kept to myself.

Things were falling into place really quickly, but we were dependent on the boys accepting what was going on and they had to pass Common Entrance exams. As it happened, they both passed with flying colours and there was a bonus of a bursary for Mark's art. Bedford School had just decided to enter the art world and Mark was to be the first art student. So, the family was all occupied within a tight local area, which meant John and Mark could be day boarders and the family would be together. Unfortunately, I would still be travelling, but it was only a daily commute down the A1 to Hatfield. I say "only" but it could be tedious. However, the family, together with Bonny the scruffy mongrel, would be anchored and that was rewarding for all of us.

Moving to a new house was not without its problems. My pension was obviously extended to the limit with the costs of a public school, and we needed a mortgage. There was also another issue I needed to address. My mother had suffered a great deal with the loss of my father and my grandma Lorton. She was lonely and it was time to increase the family even further. Such a move was going to be beneficial for all of us. Years before, I had helped my parents by contributing to the cost of the roof of their property. It was easy for my mother to agree to sell her small bungalow and help finance the house for the whole family. Lonely she may have been, but she still wanted some independence. I was understanding and, as luck would have it, we had a plan. There was a stable in the back garden of the new house and it was just ten yards from our backdoor. The stable was converted, a conservatory added, and that was more than satisfactory. Of course, it was all a big outlay, but Trish and I had the prospect of good jobs, which put the icing on the cake.

While the cake was being consumed, a bolt came out of the blue. On 19 October 1987, I went to Zurich.[3] On the journey home after the project meeting, I was sitting in a first-class seat and was handed a copy of *The Financial Times*. It was Black Monday! Computers had failed and there had been a dramatic fall on the stock markets, which held my recently commuted pension. I made some quick calculations and found I had lost £35,000. I asked the hostess for some champagne and got drunk.[4]

Trish was finally signed up as a PE and English teacher at Sandy Secondary School, where she was to make more-permanent friendships and to find pleasure in teaching again. There was a mountain of work ahead, but I felt contentment and peace in the family. Trish smiled again, and it was as though we had remarried. It was clear, from this moment on, that she did not want to risk harming her marriage or relationship with her family. I was quite certain the decision that had tortured me in London was the best that could have been made.

---

3 I was travelling all over Europe for meetings for BAE. I can't remember what this one was about, but I certainly remember the stock market crash.

4 As it turned out, patience was rewarded. By 1990 I had recovered my pension. So, life went on quite happily. I was lucky with the timing of events.

My new job was about an hour's drive down the A1 to the BAE Dynamics Division at Hatfield. I knew I would have to do some commuting, but the journey did not seem too bad. There was the compensation that I had treated myself to a bright red four-by-four Ford Sierra with a top speed of 150 miles per hour. It was a miracle I did not collect points and fines, especially because I had the childish thought that it had replaced the BAE Lightning with its powerful engines and reheats!

That first morning, as I parked in front of a low scruffy building, opened the front door and walked in, I felt a strange feeling of coming home. I remembered those twenty years before when I displayed with two other pilots in our Vampires at a Hatfield open day. At the time, we had been well looked after because the Vampire had started its life at Hatfield and, at the end of that day, I was given a black-and-white photo of us doing a perfect fan break over the top of a Moth and it was the Tiger Moth that I had first flown solo. I have treasured the photo ever since.

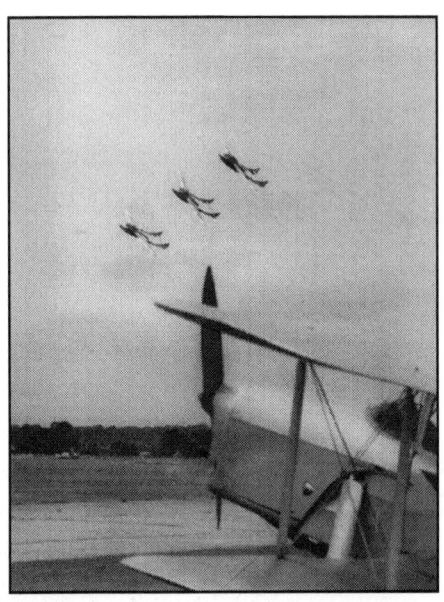

Participating with two other pilots in our Vampires at a Hatfield Open Day. Beneath is the Tiger Moth in which I first flew solo.

My role at Hatfield was as Manager of Weapon Concepts. I entered a small department with about ten others. I found myself in charge of this small unit, which was part of BAE Operational Analysis, which at that stage was spread across the company. There were similar small departments spread across Dynamics specialising in ground-to-air at Stevenage, special weapons at Bristol and air-to-air and air-to-ground at Hatfield. Preston had a bigger department to cover aircraft production, but the clever stuff was undoubtedly about the weapons. The people at Hatfield were researchers and programmers but my job, with another ex-RAF officer, was to work on the concept of use. I was soon promoted to Head of Operational Assessment.

There were some key players; they had deep expertise that was beyond my experience, and I was going to have to rely on them. Rob Whittaker was the most experienced analyst. He was closely supported by Jenny Young, who was also young and clever, and I certainly needed their technical judgement. Soon to follow me was Squadron Leader Graham Thompson, who was ex-RAF and complementary to me and understood more about air-to-ground weapons. Stuck in a corner reading was Ros Howell, an ex-Air Defence controller. I was to learn she was highly intelligent but at this stage had no particular role. Around and about were several specialist assistant analysts and computer administrators. Somewhere across the site was an executive-in-charge. That was Air Commodore John Mitchell and he too had been a Lightning pilot and I had known him over the years.

As my first day ended, I realised that, more than anything, I had to bring the analysts together as a team and understand the people and their work. Just before we packed up on that first day, I gathered them together and said, "You may think my request is somewhat strange, but would the first person in the office on future mornings put the kettle on for coffee and tea and, for a few minutes each day, we will exchange absolutely any thoughts."[5] It was a simple request, but it was to bear fruit.

The day over, I jumped into my red racer and headed north, but I realised I had found out only a little about my future professional life. Yet again, I was going to have to get used to keeping my life in separate compartments. For outside work you do not gain popularity by declaring you have a job thinking about killing people and causing maximum destruction with clever technology. However, at five o'clock (not 1700 hours) I could go home and be with my family and enter the other compartment.

---

5   Later, after the Covid pandemic, there was a policy of working from home (WFH). If it had happened in my time at Hatfield, progress would have suffered. Only later was I to realise my timing as Head of Operational Assessment was lucky.

Chapter Two
Windsurfing

The family soon settled into a new routine. I was pleased Trish made firm friends with her fellow teachers. John was not impressed with Bedford School; he was just eager to get through school and get on with adult life, much as I had been in my teenage years. It was good to have him around the house because he was becoming big and strong and helpful with heavy tasks. Mark just got on with his art, setting his own standards at Bedford School, which included a mohican haircut! Trish and I were called to Bedford and requested to influence Mark's standard of dress. In the end, Bedford School had gone down the artistic route and differences from the norm were tolerated. In retrospect, that freedom was to help him develop and get a first at Covent Garden.

Both Tina and Lesley had boyfriends and Tina was to head off to India on a long holiday with her boyfriend after finishing her degree course. Lesley was very young and wanted to settle with a young man in Devon. Trish and I were not impressed with either, but I agreed with Trish that we should let them find their own way. What we wanted was to ensure that our communication with them was to remain uncomplicated. I remembered my early love life and realised that if parents interfered it could cause a lifetime of difficulty. I remember Trish's mother in the same difficult situation saying, "You make your bed, you lie on it."

She had obviously come to the same conclusion and was concerned about what her daughter was doing.[6]

Just as we had settled into our new life, John arrived home from school one evening, after he had been out with the Combined Cadet Force (CCF) to a flooded quarry in Woodhall Spa, with a request that was to change our family's life.

"Dad, I've been having a go at windsurfing. It was fun. When we were finished, we were offered windsurfer boards and rigs at a cheap price. What do you think?"

It was still early days for this new sport. I knew it existed but not much about it.

I replied, "I have done a lot of sailing in different boats, and it can't be much different, so let's have a go."

Trish was listening and was wincing. I knew what

---

[6] A strange thought entered my head. Trish and I overcame the resistance to our marrying because we were too young. When I married Mary, her son did not like the idea that I was old. However, as I write, I have managed to keep my marriages intact for sixty-five years. I am proud of that.

she was thinking: *Here we go again. The bugger is going to disappear over the horizon and this time he's going to take my son with him.*

Things got even more complicated when Mark said, "Me too."

I replied, "Mark, of course you can join in, but let John and me understand what it's all about and then we can help you. I will also have to understand something about the cost before we fling ourselves in the deep end."

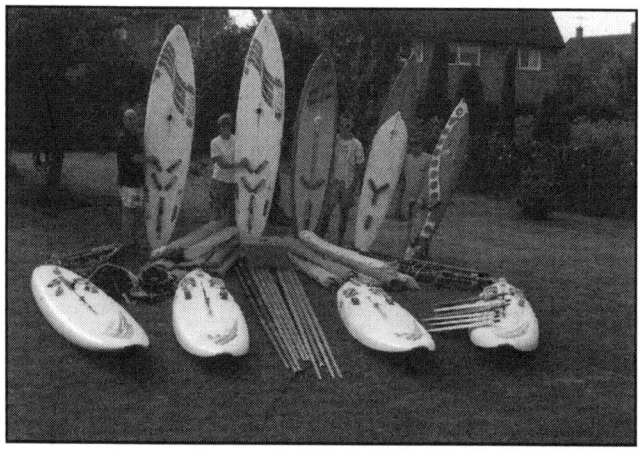

With our first surfboards in the back garden of our house in Gamlingay (from left to right: me, Trish, John, Mark)

It was also in my mind that, at thirteen years old, Mark had a great sense of balance, but needed time to grow a bit more. I still recalled that I had built an Oppy (children's racing dinghy) for John and Mark, and Mark had abandoned it on launching it into the

Malacca Straits and swum home. We had to send a boat out to recover it. Meanwhile, Trish's face was looking skywards in despair. I was waiting for the outburst, and it came very quickly.

"You men are not going to do this to me. This time I'm coming with you. I'm going to have some fun too."

I knew Trish was capable; she was a PE teacher, physically fit and a really good swimmer with no fear of the water. In big boats she had been seasick but being active on a small board would probably cure that problem. I was so pleased Trish was onside. The decision was made. We were going to be a windsurfing family, whatever that meant. I ordered a Mistral windsurfing board. It was to be the first of many.

Things were settling into a pattern, but I had to get a grip on my work at Hatfield. Tea on arrival turned out to be a brilliant idea. I just let the morning salutations drift into the weather and general conversation, and then one analyst would ask how things were going and the conversation drifted into problem-solving. In the main, I just listened and learnt. At this stage, all the work was involved with air-to-air and air-to-ground weapons but as the months passed this was to change. Our tasks looked at anti-radar and short- and beyond-visual-range air-fighting missiles. We looked at sensors, war heads, energy and manoeuvrability, and sensors in aircraft. Analysis was not limited to BAE products, and comparisons were made with Soviet and NATO equipment. It was an interesting task. The Soviet Union was also coming to its end, and I was participating in think tanks about changes at the Royal Institute of International Affairs and the Royal United Services Institute.[7]

The first windsurfing board was delivered, and we joined Grafham Water Sailing Club. I said to John, "I've been a sailing instructor, and it can't be much different to sailing a dinghy."

So, we went to Grafham and Trish and Mark watched our puny attempts. We learnt to balance and sail in a straight line, but to turn round meant entering the water one way or another. To gybe was impossible because I was insisting on gybing as in a sailing boat. On a windsurfer this was a duck gybe which was a gybe done by top experts. It was entirely different from sailing a dinghy and, in the end, we found a lady instructor to teach us the fundamentals. Our eyes were opened. As winter approached, we bought wetsuits and we improved with some moderate success. Along came a second board and Mark started jumping up and down for his turn.

So, my initial thought of dinghy sailing started to

---

[7] The first is famous for its Chatham House papers covering wide political issues. The second is very much about conflict. I was a member of RUSI for some years. Prince Philip tried to give members defence knowledge recognition and degrees, much as happens in the USA. I think our education authorities were against the idea.

take a back seat and the family enthusiasm became a united enthusiasm for windsurfing.

By March 1985, John and I became over-confident and declared we would become competitive and go racing. It was still icy cold and there was a force 5 wind when we entered the Round Mersea Island Race. It was also early days for windsurfing technology. Everything was heavy; it was difficult to find the centre of balance and such old kit was unforgiving. We spent time recovering our cold bodies from the water and the procedure was exhausting. To enter a race with so many competitors, all coping with their own problems, increased the need for us to raise our skills to another level. There was chaos, and the chaos caused one false start after another. The wetsuits let in the icy water and our hands froze. Once our hands became numb, our brains followed, and we entered the water even more. An hour went by, and we made a start, but I was finished. I sailed for the shore exhausted and close to hypothermia; I felt disconsolate. John was obviously having success, but no! Further along the shore I could see a windsurfer in a similar state. It was John. The whole event could have been the end of competitive windsurfing but there was something in our genes that increased our determination. We were going to rise to the challenge.

Mark was still jumping up and down, only restrained by Trish demanding warmer weather for both. The family was becoming bound together and obsessed with windsurfing. It was not just the windsurfing binding us together, but also our total lifestyle as a family. In the morning, we would always get up and head off for the day. The boys and Trish went to school. Mark always had difficulty raising his head out of bed and there was frustration from Trish who was trying to meet a morning driving schedule. I generally left earlier to get down the A1 to Hatfield. In other words, we were just a normal family with the boys whining and reluctantly making their way to school, as would be expected of teenagers. At home we were all working to renovate the granny annexe and again we worked as a team. Up went a garden room on the outside of the annexe; up went fences; and the sheds were readied for our new sport.

We were soon all set for our new life. The annexe was soon renovated, and my mother moved in. I think the building itself was OK and she never complained, but something was wrong. It was as though a light had gone out. She shut the door and isolated herself. She would rarely come the ten yards to our backdoor, and she had an unbreakable routine. We could go for coffee at eleven o'clock, but it had to be to time, otherwise, it would not happen. She had her TV programmes, and they were sacrosanct. However, she never complained; she just existed. She had spent her whole life with Sam in business and at home, and she had lost him. She had cared for him and my grandmother, both of whom had died of cancer at the same time, and she just waited for the end. Only now, as I am immersed in my final years, do I have an inkling of what she must have been going through. It must have been hell for her. Sometimes I just wish I had done more. I was her only child and had spent my life on another planet with my own problems that had been kept hidden from her.

We were now set up for the next five years. There was time for the boys to finish their secondary education, Trish would have a settled job, and my job would develop. Mum would remain hidden from the cruel world. Above all, there was windsurfing.

With the arrival of the first summer, much time was spent at Grafham Water Sailing Club and all four family members progressed. Suppertime at home was all about wind strength, tacking, gybing and water starting. The boys' progress, as expected, was at a phenomenal rate; Mum and Dad followed more slowly. Our family was not alone. It was a time when windsurfing as a sport was exploding and equipment developed to make progress a little easier.

The club had been hit quite badly by a recession, but as the windsurfer numbers increased, so the club was pulled away from financial problems. However, there was resentment. The older sailing fraternity really did not like these upstarts on the same waters but realised they were a necessary evil. As I improved, the whole club accepted me because of my wider sailing knowledge. I became Windsurfing Fleet Captain and took my place on the club committee. Slowly, the racing fleets tolerated the windsurfers racing in their own fleet and, on occasions, with them. Eventually, I became Vice Commodore with the right to become Commodore. I sensed the fear of my right to become Commodore, especially as the windsurfing voting strength was dominant, and realised I had gone as far as I should go. That was the end of my authority in the club as a whole. I resigned in order to keep the peace and let the "yachties" have their club back, but the club recognised a change had taken place and there was acceptance of the change, which was good. I then turned my attention to honing my skills; John and I became RYA instructors and Trish got a qualification to teach children, which fitted in with her PE teaching role. John also supported the local shop by teaching customers. I later took a long course with the RYA and became a race coach. The family made lots of friends and we had a base for our windsurfing from where we were to roam widely, both at leisure and in racing competitions. It was an engrossing lifestyle.

Windsurfing competitiveness developed along two paths. One was all raceboard racing along similar lines to dinghy racing. The longboard was standardized with a centreboard, and in the 1980s, the sail size was limited to 7.5 square metres. It was all amateur; the route to the Olympics and our British organisation was the UKBSA (UK Board Sailing Association). The other path was shortboard sailing, in the British Funboard Association (BFA). The competitions in the BFA could be wave, speed, slalom or longboard. Because the boards were small, sailing normally took place in a force 4 wind or above. It was the route to professional competition because it was more spectacular. At this stage another organisation was forming for thirty-five-year-olds and above, known as Seavets.

Initially, John, Mark and I joined both the UKBSA and BFA, although we favoured the BFA. It was the right place to go for the boys because the sailing was strenuous and more exciting for those in early manhood. I was in my late forties and it was very challenging for me, but I wanted to sail with my boys. I could sail in the senior section for the over-thirty-fives, but even in that section the competition was tough. However, it was too late for me to compete in the waves, and I stuck to course- and slalom-racing mainly on small boards. So it was that we all sailed at every opportunity, either by travelling to a national competition or in club racing. Trish sailed when the weather was kind enough and mainly at Grafham. She was making friends and eyeing up the Seavets, which she joined later. We all became very lean and fit, and it certainly helped me throw off the stress of the early 1980s. The obsession was expensive but we did get some sponsorship as a family, from Mistral, which helped with the cost of equipment. However, the main cost was travel and accommodation. In later years I was to tell the boys there was no money in windsurfing and, if they were to have a family, to enjoy windsurfing as a leisure activity but to stay away from competition for it could be horrendously expensive. However, John and his children were not to heed my advice.

Of course, I did not follow my own advice. While the boys progressed easily and took to high winds, small boards and the waves, for me it was dogged hard work but I was, as ever, determined to get my piece of the action. At the BFA and once out to sea there were usually several races before we came back ashore. The races were always in high winds and around the same course, usually about an hour long. In the main, we took our results in the group we were sailing in. Eventually, Mark settled in the youths, John amongst the professionals, and I was in the seniors. At the worst stage of my windsurfing career, I would be more in the water than on it and would end the race way last and exhausted. I was one of the oldest competitors and the least experienced. I would finish the race and then, as I crossed the line, the five-minute gun would go for the next start. The whole fleet was well rested except for me. I crossed the start line of the second and third races in complete exhaustion. After four or five hours at sea, I would crawl up the shingle, drink gallons of tea and fall asleep while the youngsters started partying. It was not long before I visited the doctors with a bad back and I was given no sympathy. I was told I was too old and should give windsurfing a miss. I found a windsurfing doctor who understood me, changed to him and pressed on.

While leisure sailing at Grafham in strong winds, Trish would worry about the boys. John was quick to give his point of view and in a frustrated voice he snapped back at Trish, "Mum, stop worrying about us. It's Dad you must worry about."

It was true but mums have an instinct to protect their sons and expect husbands to know their limitations. Wrong!

When I thought I was beginning to progress and we were coming out of winter, the first race at Marazion in Cornwall was to become a memorable disaster. I still had a lot to learn.

It was windy, very windy, and the waves breaking into the beach were way beyond my capability and beyond the capability of most of the seniors. Nevertheless, I put together a small kit to make my way out to go slalom racing. As I stood in the water with my board and sail held high and the hope that I could throw it down and jump on it at a calm moment between waves, I looked ahead at the wall of water and knew this was going to be difficult. To my amazement, I got the timing right and was on my way over set after set of waves, and then I was clear and out in the open sea.

However, I must have relaxed too much and hit a big rogue wave and was then flattened by a gust of wind. The board flew into the air and was lost to me. Suddenly I felt lonely, and it was going to be a long swim back through the breaking waves. I got through the first breaking wave, then things started to get really difficult. The next wave was big, and I was losing energy. I swam to the top of the wave but, as it broke, I fell into the undertow and was dragged back underwater. I swam as hard as I could to get to the surface, but when I got to the top of the wave the whole process was repeated; each time I did this I was getting short of oxygen.

In the middle of the wave sets, I really thought I was going to drown. When I got my head above water, I could see a beautiful sight. It was a fellow windsurfer about to launch into the surf. For the first and only time in my life, I shouted for help. I bellowed and anyone who knows me knows I can bellow. The windsurfer's body straightened, and I could see his head searching. Then he jumped on his board and headed out. He was going to help me. Then I saw him fly into the air off a wave and he departed from his board. That was the last I saw of my would-be helper, and it was back to the washing machine for me, but I was learning.

If I could not outswim the undertow, I could find my way out of the top of the wave and avoid it breaking. This gave me time to breathe, and I stopped panicking. I then picked my waves and made progress. I eventually lay on the shingle, completely devoid of energy. I slowly recovered. I could not see my helper and never did find him. I presume he, like me, searched along the shore looking for his board. He must have found his board, seen me upwind and gone home. I de-rigged my battered kit and returned to the motorhome.

"Good sail?" asked Trish. "Would you like a cup of tea?"

"Yes, please," I replied. "That would be nice."

Later that day I told her I had not raced because I thought the weather was too much.

"At last, Terry, you're acting your age."

As time passed, I told her the truth and admitted that, yet again, I had been very lucky.

I was not the only one in the family that had exciting moments; all of us had interesting times.

Quite early on, Mark was trying to do tricks on

Grafham Water on a small board, which was quite difficult without proper waves. Nevertheless, he was keen to be the first at doing a loop. One day he arrived back ashore in cold, windy conditions to tell everyone he had "done it", but no one had seen him. He said he had hurt his wrist, but he would go out again and prove it. Well, he did it again but when his arm warmed up he was in pain. He had broken a bone!

Later, John and Mark settled into a routine of jumping and looping and whatever went with the fashion. If I got airborne on a wave, it was a mistake. It was too late in my life to get water starts in huge waves; that was for the young braves. Trish remained on flat water and race boards. When she had trouble, she had three menfolk to rescue her and bring her home.

I had been to hospital after head-butting the mast, but one day I really feared for John. I thought we had lost him.

When we were all competent, we decided to go to Lanzarote. We had a deal where we could transport all our own kit at little cost. We spent days packing five boards and goodness knows how many sails and paraphernalia into bubble wrap. When we booked in at the airport, we had four trolleys connected in a line. We were a spectacle and gathered a crowd.

We were set up for a fantastic holiday but there

were problems. The winds and waves could be quite demanding, and the first thing to go was Mark's beloved Krakatoa custom board, which broke in half. Tears flowed and calm only fell on the family after we had bought a similar board from the local professional. The problem was that this was badly designed and was not in the same category as the beloved Krakatoa.

We all had knocks and bangs. I had to have coral removed from my foot.

But one day, there was a strong offshore wind and John had only hired a small board. I saw John go down in the distance and he did not come up. Things were serious! Trish went into a panic and, although I reassured her, I was beginning to panic too. There were no rescue facilities on Lanzarote, and I ran up and down the coast looking for a motorboat, or police, or any help I could find. I was generally greeted with a shrug and a language problem. In any case, I had long since learnt that motorboats do not go out in strong offshore winds. There was no help to be found. It was a long way from Lanzarote to West Africa.

Just when my panic was at its peak, I thought I saw a sail on the horizon and yes, it was *his* sail! It was heading well downwind of his starting point.

I eventually found John on the beach. He was hunched up, with his arms round his knees and looking out to sea. He did not want to talk but just kept looking out to the horizon. He had fought his own battle, much as I had done at Marazion, and knew it had been a close call.

The French BIC board was known to be delicate. In the heaving sea, the small track that had held the universal and sail together had broken in half, and half had disappeared. It required extraordinary effort from John not to lose either the board or sail. Somehow or other, he managed to hold the board on its side in the heaving waves and to thread a small nut and bolt into the remaining track. It is the sort of task, when everything is moving about, that needs three hands. It took him a long time and, all the time, he was being blown farther from land. No wonder I found him hunched up, exhausted and speechless.

Not that Trish was without her windsurfing excitement. The incident I will relate here was serious.

We often visited Portland to sail and would launch from the marina at the entry point to the causeway between Weymouth and Portland. It was during one of two spring tides that year that Trish and I decided to leave the Portland area on long boards and sail across the harbour into Weymouth Bay. There was a force 4 wind. We first sailed to windward to reach Weymouth, then turned round and planed back and forth downwind towards the marina.

As I came ashore, I expected Trish to come ashore

with me, but she was nowhere in sight. I rushed back to our motorhome and got a pair of binoculars. I started to get worried, but the binoculars solved the problem, and I could see her. She was quite far out to sea and seemed to be kneeling on the water. It was all quite strange, until I remembered it was an exceptionally low tide and there was a sandbank well out into the harbour. However, this was only a problem twice a year.

I told people what I was going to do and sailed out to her. She was now lying on her back and could not stand up. The water there was extremely shallow, and she had hit the bank at speed. I unzipped the wetsuit leg and could see straight away her ankle was broken.

"It's OK, Trish. I think you've sprained your ankle," I lied. "I'll have to get you ashore."

"Oh, that's good. I thought I might have broken it," she said.

Now, getting Trish ashore was a problem. The shortest way was to some rocks but that was going to be difficult. I forgot the boards, but luckily, I was being watched through binoculars and some young guys were beginning to realise they could help. I picked Trish up and walked across the sandbar, but the water then came up to my chest and progress through the seaweed was not easy. I knew that when I got her to the rocks, I would need help. There was no way I could get her over seaweed and rocks by myself. So, after I had got her safely out of the water, I told her I would have to get help. I climbed over the rocks and onto the road and started running. I must have run about half a mile in the wetsuit before I found a phone box (yes, it was in the days of phone boxes). I dialled 999, gasping for air, and explained the situation. I began to realise how far I had run because paramedics reached Trish at the same time as I arrived back. I gave her a kiss and said I would be with her as soon as I could. When I got back to the marina the boards had been collected and de-rigged. I was so grateful for the help and, in no time at all, I was on my way to the hospital.

Trish had been planing when she hit the bank and her foot had dragged her toe back and split the bone up through the ankle. Not a good break. When the doctor saw her, he told her that, at her age, it was the end of her windsurfing. Much as in my discussion with the doctor about hurting my back years before, Trish politely disagreed, and she joined the Seavets and windsurfed for many years after. It seemed determination (or was it bloody-mindedness?) was now endemic in the family.

Of course, rescuing was not all one-sided and in the family. As my experience increased, I made numerous rescues of others, but one stood out for Trish and me when we were at Tarifa in southern Spain. Tarifa is something of a mecca of waves and windsurfing and I was at the height of my ability. The year was 2002.

I carried out a rescue and sent an e-mail home. It read thus:

What you will need to understand is that I reckon that I am the oldest Englishman sailing out here at the moment, although there is a Belgian and a German that are both older and there is a tale to tell about the Belgian, who is incredibly stoic. He is now sixty-seven and six years ago he collided with a German in the surf and broke his leg in three places. Four years later he got prostate cancer badly but was back windsurfing at the end of the year. And last year he had a heart attack in the surf and went back to hospital again for six bypasses. He is back again this year but windsurfing and surfing with a little caution.

I do not even start to match his bravery, but slowly I have once again got into the Tarifa windsurfing scene, and I am probably watched by some of the younger generation with a little interest. I realise I look somewhat quaint wearing my old lifejacket and helmet, come what may.

On the day in question, the "problem" of my age became a slight issue. The Levant (easterly wind) had set in early and was forecast to be force 4 inshore and force 5 outside. In Tarifa terms, this is regarded as a light wind. I elected to take my AHD 65 out and a six-metre sail. The board was big, but the sail was spot on, and I had real wild sailing on building seas. About three o'clock, Trish joined me on the beach, and I said I was beginning to get a bit tired and would have one more session and then stop. (It was 13 Feb.) By now I had been joined by quite a number of sailors, mostly on wave boards and 5.5-metre sails. I sailed quite a long way out because the Levant was receding out to sea. As I was about to enter a gybe, I could see one of these wave boards even further out and there was something strange about it. I went out to investigate.

When I got there, the wave sailor was trying to tow another sailor on his board ... with little success. When they both flopped into the water, I gybed and settled alongside the two of them. The windsurfer in distress had broken his mast and had to ditch his rig. We were a long way out and the seas were not insignificant for the task of getting home.

The sailors were young men and the one in distress, as I was to learn later, was called Elsor. He was in his mid-twenties, and he weighed ninety-two kilograms! After a short while, I suggested that perhaps I could be of help. Elsor was not rude but, when he got close enough, he could see the wrinkles in my face and he said he would be happier for both of us if someone more youthful rescued him.

Unfortunately for this argument, his would-be rescuer then came clean and said he could not cope with his kit. I then suggested that they should take my kit and tow me in, but that was also declined. We then discussed the likelihood of a rescue boat arriving and we agreed that there was no rescue boat on shore, and it would take a long time to alert any rescue services, especially as we were so far out (two miles or more). Eventually the conversation ran out of steam, and they started to look at the Old Man in the Sea for some sort of solution. I then went through a very short interview, which consisted of the question, "Have you done much windsurfing?" to which I answered, "My wife thinks I do rather a lot." I was now hired.

I asked the other young man to sail home and alert Club Mistral (from whence they had come) and I would do my best to tow Elsor back. It was now that my bigger board and bigger sail came into their own. Even though the sea was moving up and down several feet, I was able to uphaul and manoeuvre with Elsor until he could grab the back of the board. He then grabbed one of the back straps and locked his other long arm round the back of my board, effectively turning it into one long board. I then powered up the sail and off we went. The strain on my arms was huge and eventually I hooked in. Wrong! The first wave just screwed us into wind and put me into the water.

I came up puffing and showing my age. I could feel what Elsor was thinking.

"OK," I said, "We will have to be patient. We'll do this in stages. The tide has turned, and we will not have to go downwind any further." There were large rocks if we came ashore downwind of our starting points. "I cannot hook in. My arms are going to get tired. We have three hours of light and people should soon know of our predicament. I will get you back. I am not going home without you."

We went through the routine of uphauling, linking up and sailing. This time I just stayed mobile on the board, putting my front foot right up on the nose of the board as we went over the top of the waves. However, after our first stop, we did not seem to put even the slightest dent in the transit home. But we got better at working together, and slowly but surely the coast got closer. As this became apparent Elsor kept saying, "Impressive. This is really impressive!"

My arms were killing me, but these few words really spurred me on. We went through the resting-and-linking procedure a couple more times and eventually we just surfed in together on the top of a small wave. What's more, I had delivered him back upwind of my own starting point, right in front of the Hurricane Hotel and Club Mistral. I sat on the beach, while there was an inquisition about the lost rig. While I listened to them, I felt totally "buggered", but pleased that the Old Man in the Sea was back home from the sea. I was offered thanks by Elsor and the Club Mistral ... but still no real rescue in sight. They asked what they could do for me. No, I didn't want a reward, just some help with my kit down the beach and the promise that someone would do the same for me one day, should I need rescuing.

Elsor carried my board down the beach and dumped it down in front of Trish, who listened to the conversation, watched the handshakes, and for a short while thought the big fellow had picked her little old fellow out of the surf. It took a short explanation to reverse the situation and I was rewarded with a big kiss and a cup of tea. You will recall that Spencer Tracy was only fed coffee.

I will also relate one incident involving Mark; he told me the story because we were alone.

Avon Beach, near Christchurch in Dorset, is a great place to sail, especially when the wind is up, but there is a tidal problem that is almost second to none. When the tide goes out there is a conflict between the race out of the harbour and the main channel stream. The result of this conflict is the current can go straight out to sea from the shore.

It is not a good thing to sail alone at nightfall, which is what Mark did and, of course, he had gear failure. It would have been a good story if it were told in the BBC programme *Saving Lives at Sea*, but there was no rescue and he had to swim home in the dark and against the adverse current. I never understood the detail, but I did realise he had had a bowel-tightening incident, probably as much as the rest of the family had experienced with their incidents.

This is an article written on Facebook by Jean Fettes of early involvement with Seavets:

In 2002, Paul (Jean's husband) and I were in Poole with the Seavets when we were invited to join Terry and Trish Adcock on their family holiday to France. This sounded a wonderful idea, so we quickly arranged our travel plans and the following month we headed across the Channel. Terry and family had travelled ahead of us. We were in their hands entirely as the campsite needed to be child friendly and very close to the beach, and we would be contacted when they had found the right place. In due course a text arrived saying they would meet us at the Camping Municipal de Penthièvre in area "L". Little did we know then that this was the start of a big adventure that would last for years. The Quiberon Peninsula is in southern Brittany. It has Quiberon Bay on the east side and the Atlantic and the Côte Sauvage on the west. Camping Municipal de Penthièvre is situated on the Bay and has direct access to the sea.

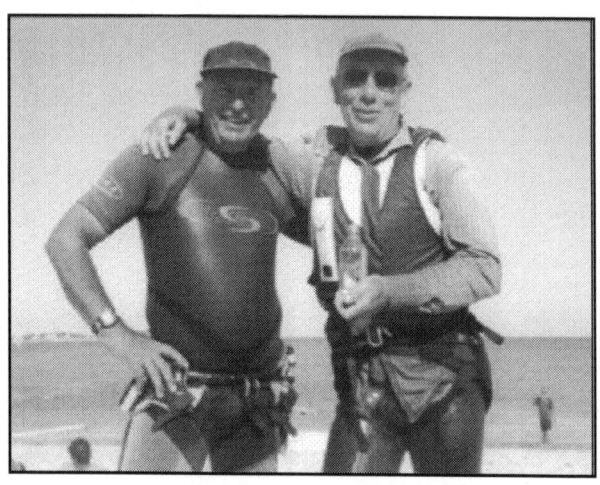

Me and Paul in Penthièvre

What a great holiday we all had. The sun shone and the wind blew. Paul and Terry were out sailing most days and the sea was super for swimming. When the tide was low (and it goes out a long way) there were plenty of other things to keep us and the kids amused. There is a summer train service, le Tire-Bouchon (the Corkscrew), which runs all day from Auray to Quiberon and back and, luckily for us, the train station is situated at the back of the campsite. Great for easy access.

Quiberon town is delightful with its seafront restaurants and small boutiques. There used to be a park in the middle with large trees providing much needed shade on a hot day, but sadly that has now been replaced by a pedestrian piazza with seating and a few new trees. Such is progress!

The Standing Stones at Carnac are a short drive or cycle ride away and well worth a visit. Just like Stonehenge you do wonder how they were all arranged there. Their name is "The Alignments" for obvious reasons, as they are all in lines, several rows abreast, from largest to smallest for about a mile. Truly amazing. There are many dolmens around the area as well.

Inland of the town of Auray, Camping Municipal de Penthièvre is situated on the Bay and has direct access to the sea. It is picturesque with its river harbour and restaurants. You can also drive or cycle along the Côte Sauvage (Wild Coast) and enjoy the wonderful scenery.

There were great evenings on site which we all enjoyed. One special last evening was when Paul and Terry went for an evening coffee and brandy (accompanied by Mo, Terry's eldest grandson) to the on-site bar. Terry was encouraged by the barman to sample some special Calvados (from an unmarked bottle!) which went straight to his head evidently, as he said to Paul, "I have to go outside in the fresh air." (They were already sitting outside.)

Then, Terry got the hiccups and the barman said, "You are hoquet," (hiccups) and Terry replied, "I am far from OK."

From then on, he has been known as Mr OK. They staggered back from the bar looking like Laurel and Hardy and it was certainly another fine mess they had got into! Mo summed it up succinctly, saying, "It was all right till they had the coffee, then it all went wrong."

All too soon our time in Penthièvre was at an end and Terry suggested that we had a group photograph. We smiled for the camera with a Seavets banner in front of us for posterity. Then he said, "This would be a great place for a Seavets holiday and as you are going to be chairman next year, Paul, you can organise it."

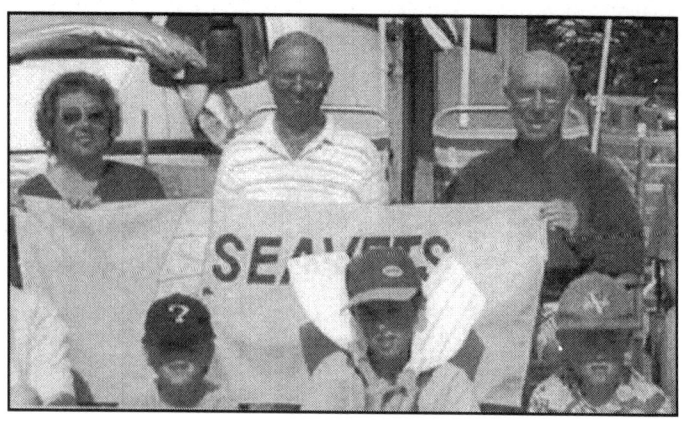

Jean and Paul Fettes with me at a Seavets holiday in Quiberon

So, we did, and the rest, as they say, is history: twenty years of it.

During the past two decades, over one hundred people have joined us in Penthièvre plus seven assorted children, twelve dogs and one cat. Sadly, we have also had our losses and we raise a glass to all our absent friends.[8]

When I eventually retired as Chairperson and windsurfing faded, I thought that would be the end of the family activity, but we now have a granddaughter, Izzy, who has been National Champion for some years and sails on a foil and competes in world competitions. She was a potential Olympic athlete until the pandemic and higher education complicated her life, but she remains a coach. Mia, Izzy's elder sister, and her partner, Rob, are also employed at the sailing centre at Portland training others. So, the seeds sown at Grafham Water all those years ago still flower.

These stories are just a few; there are many more that could be told. What windsurfing did was to bind the family together for many years. In competitions, John and Mark won accolades at national level and for one year I managed to get my act together to become Senior National Champion. Trish and I joined the Seavets when we retired. That is where ageing windsurfers go to race and socialise, and I became

---

8 Written by Jean Fettes looking back to the beginning of Seavets' visits to Quiberon.

Chairperson for a number of years. When we retired, we both thought that would be that, but we had a granddaughter who became National Champion and fourth in the world at the age of fifteen, but she gave it up to concentrate on her career. However, water sports just got into the family's blood and remained there.

Chapter Three
Hatfield, Computers and the SDI

Although the house, family and windsurfing were now driving my life, I still had to go to work, and it was a case of up and down the A1 to and from Hatfield each day. I shared the driving with Cliff Downs who also lived in Gamlingay and managed the computer systems at BAE Systems. We were later joined in the travelling by his son, Simon, who worked for me on the unit database.

Strange things seem to happen time and again in my life. A day or two after I had written Simon's name, having not seen him for over thirty years, the phone rang and it was Simon. He had found out where I was living and wanted to visit with his wife, Chris. Why, after all this time, remained a mystery because I could remember little about all the staff. I think the trigger may have been his meeting a Lightning enthusiast in a pub and Simon mentioned he had worked for me. He had said to Simon that Simon had worked for a Lightning legend. It was very embarrassing listening to the story, but the outcome was that Simon and Chris turned up on Easter Saturday and we had lunch together. They arrived with chocolates and flowers and Simon immediately said he had come to say thank you.

Thank you for what? I thought.

He explained that I had given him his first job and it had been one of the most enjoyable. But most of all, it had set him off on a successful career. He told me stories about the people in the department and said I had also taken him windsurfing with John and Mark, but the most interesting story I had completely forgotten.

I had forgotten that when I left the RAF, I had bought a flame-red Ford Sierra 4 Sri. I was driving down the A1 when Simon asked how hot the car was. I knew it would get from zero to sixty in seven seconds and no one saw me off from the lights, but I had never tested the top speed. Well, the road was absolutely clear, and Simon told me we hit 142 miles per hour. I guess as a young person, and probably petrified, he had good reason to remember.

As he told the story I started to remember, but I looked across to Mary, who was listening, and realised my cover was blown. Her jaw had dropped because I made it a big issue that I always obeyed the law because a good driver drove accurately, not showing off at great speed. Anyway, he had asked. Simon also recalled that Mark had a reputation for always insisting on stopping at a Little Chef to eat a burger. Did he still enjoy them? I smiled and told him that Mark would be horrified, for he was now a committed vegan. My driving and Mark's diet had turned 180 degrees since those days. It is good to have someone tell you about your own past.

Cliff worked in a different department and as a computer expert. It was a good arrangement to travel with them because I was to be in charge of experts working in Operational Assessment and if I was confused by their technology I could learn from Cliff on our travels. I was also gaining hands-on experience with a computer at home. It was the era of the Sinclair ZX Spectrum into which software was loaded off cassette tape. It took ages to start up and load a programme, but it served its purpose and I started to understand programming even in machine code. Cliff had a BBC Acorn, which seemed to be much more upmarket, and BASIC software programming came onto the scene and slowly things became easier. It was in the mid-eighties that computer development exploded, especially on the desktop. IBM, the biggest company in the world, stuck with mainframe development and lost out to the likes of Apple and Microsoft. While my task was to understand developing intelligence threats and the use of weapons, playing around with computing helped me to understand something about the tools of the trade of my staff. Together we could develop computer models to establish the way forward for weapon development. Sadly, Cliff died not many years after our association.

As I write this, I have picked up my work notes and tried to understand what was going on, but not being a mathematician or physicist—and with the passage of the years—it is impossible to decode them. Did I even understand at the time? Perhaps I did not have to understand, because there were experts around me and all I had to understand was the effect of developing technology and, in particular, where the Soviet Union and other areas in the world stood with regard to that technology. It was the time of Ronald Reagan and his Strategic Defense Initiative (Star Wars) and his need to use the best brains he could find in the Western world. Of course, some of those brains were in the UK and BAE and there were dollar-led contracts floating around. I started to attend presentations from intelligence organisations and technology companies about the effects of the change from mutual assured destruction (MAD) to the defence of the strategic nuclear threat in space. It was heady stuff about directed energy weapons (DEW), non-nuclear electromagnetic pulse (N^2EMP) weapons, rail guns and the like. It was a clever Cold War policy because the Soviet Union had to follow at a time when their politics and economy were under great stress. Whether it actually brought down the Soviet Union is open to debate, but it certainly helped to destroy their economy, on which their weapon development depended. The spin-off of such electromagnetic research has since been incorporated into weapon production within the earth's atmosphere.

Apart from the esoteric stuff, there was the production of more down-to-earth weapons and, right at the start of my new job, I became involved in the design and upgrade of Sea Eagle, a stand-off anti-ship weapon, and I realised that coincidence had caused my involvement in weapon design in the previous decade—the early seventies—when I was on the staff of the admiral in charge of the Second Flotilla, Rear Admiral Richard Clayton. We had finished an exercise and I reported to him that the RN could no longer be satisfied with helicopters firing wire-guided missiles at ships. The idea that a helicopter could rise high enough to fire a missile inside ships' defences and stay still during the whole process was suicidal for the helicopters and the time had come to purchase fire-and-forget weapons which were fired from sea level. Admiral Clayton told me to draft a case for a new weapon, which he signed off. A decade later the weapon had been fitted to the Buccaneer (fixed-wing attack aircraft on the aircraft carriers at the time) and to the Lynx helicopter, and almost my first task was to help with an upgrade and sales.

My staff for this and other tasks consisted of two

main departments: a conceptual group of ex-RAF operators headed by Peter Barnett and a group involved with battle analysis. The latter encompassed a smaller group involved with detailed engagement analysis and was headed up by Rob Whitaker.

Technology, business and administrative support were also embedded within the groups. Apart from managing the operational assessment, I would also get deeply involved with the trials of air-to-air and air-to-ground weapons and the sensitivity of intelligence and emerging technology. The former would bring me into close contact with another pilot, Graham Thompson, and the latter was an ex-Air Defence controller, Ros Howell. The whole outfit became very close and at the start of the day, as people arrived at work, we would settle as usual around a teapot and talk.

Some parts of the work were fun. Graham and I would go to BAE Wharton with some of the analysts. There we would "fly" profiles in different aircraft with different missiles. The chief analyst was Rob Whitaker and once again I was lucky to have a brilliant mind alongside. Not only was he a clever scientist but also—what was important to me—was the fact he developed good relationships with his staff and got the very best out of them. We would mix up US, Soviet and British aircraft and missiles and feed the results into missiles being developed in the USA for

USAF and RAF. In the main, we were looking at the development of the advanced short-range air-to-air missile (ASRAAM) and the advanced medium-range air-to-air missile (AMRAAM), the latter being beyond visual range (BVR)—a particularly skilful profile using supersonic speeds and manoeuvrability to run the opposing threatening missile out of energy.

The reason we went to Wharton was because the Aircraft Division had two huge completely spherical domes with proper ejection seats and aircraft controls located in the middle of the spheres. Graham and I would strap into the seats with flying controls and air-to-air radars in front of us, and we would "fight to the death" with profiles fed into the radar and the "sky" from computers located elsewhere. For the short-range and visual combat clouds, the sky, the ground and the opposing aircraft were projected in CGI onto the inside of the dome. As the manoeuvres built up in the fight, the air pressure was fed into G suits round our legs to simulate the G force. It was all very realistic, hence the fun. In addition to the missile development, we were also developing helmets so we could look and shoot and increase missile capability to fire, not only at aircraft ahead, but also beyond the ninety-degree position. This was 1985 and, needless to say, it was highly classified. Today this type of war gaming is old hat, but if my sons could have seen what we were doing then they would have been amazed.

Most of our work was to do with air-launched weapons but our sister Operational Assessment Department at Bristol was working on advanced technology, and they would involve us in some of their development because of our operational experience and concept work. Well, rail gun development was interesting enough with projectiles predicted to travel at something like fifteen kilometres per second but what fascinated me was N^2EMP, which could pose an awkward threat to modern aircraft. It all started with an initial brief from a physicist called Dr David Morgan. It was well understood that the force of a nuclear explosion would be preceded by an electromagnetic pulse that would close down communications, but this was a by-product of devastation and MAD. What if the pulse could be produced without the use of a nuclear weapon? And even better, to make the single pulse "ring" for a longer time? Then, such a device could be used aggressively to close down communications in conventional war. The scientists wanted to know from us how it could be used *by* us, and—more importantly—how it could be used *against* us. The first problem was, therefore, to learn how to protect ourselves.[9] This was not an easy question to answer, especially as computing was rapidly finding its way into everyday life.

---

[9] As I write, the Russian Special Operation is not in a good place and I am surprised N2EMP has not been used. Or has it?

When I arrived at Hatfield and started to get to know my staff, there was one person sitting in the corner doing nothing in particular other than reading magazines. This was Ros Howell. She impressed me with her knowledge and intellect, and I started to give her networking tasks that led to information-gathering in the MOD and disseminating information to journalists. Through her endeavours we slowly gathered information on the way ahead, especially with the use of new technology, SDI and drones. Unfortunately, BAE saw the use of drones as being a bit juvenile and the Aircraft Division scoffed at the idea of using a "model aircraft" when they could build the real thing. What we were suggesting was way ahead of its time and Britain let the USA and other countries take the lead.

A big event came when we started to learn about the break-up of the Soviet Union. I was the BAE member on the Study of the Soviet Union at the Royal Institute of International Affairs, and we were trying to understand the quite dramatic changes in the culture and economy of the Soviet Union. At that time, Ros was networking around the same issue; she was quite sure the Soviet Union was going to fall. So, Ros drafted a paper suggesting a likely break-up and the effect it would have on BAE business. It was hard for BAE to take in because it was so dramatic, but history was to prove us right. This work was causing BAE management to sit up and take notice of our small unit, and there was a move for the Aircraft Division at Preston to put their OA manager in charge of all three OA units at Hatfield, Bristol and Stevenage. Rumours went around for some while and morale was affected because of the fear of redundancies.

Eventually, I called a meeting and asked the staff if they would support me in making a move to take charge of all OA in BAE Dynamics and I got unanimous support. This took higher management by surprise, and I think there was some fear of the Aircraft Division taking over a hostile situation. But I had my way, and all Dynamics OA was merged under my control. The RAF had taught me not to sit back and be used as a pawn.

Chapter Four
Stevenage and Recession

At my start in the BAE Dynamics Division there were 15,000 people and, while I was at Hatfield, business was booming, and manpower slowly increased to 25,000. However, there was a recession and the Soviet threat decreased and BAE started paying out redundancy for people to leave. During the cost-cutting process, OA moved to Stevenage, and I became a marketing executive working for a delightful man, Sir Alec Morris, who was an air marshal and had been Chief Engineer in the RAF, but I still had direct responsibility for operational assessment.

The whole momentum in the division was of panic and movement towards cost-cutting and marketing; I was given the task of writing a business plan for Dynamics. At the same time, I was sent on a course at the London Business School. I did not stay on the course because I could not afford the time, but I was on and off the course for periods of a few days at a time and the odd week or so. The interesting part of the course for me was to learn some of the psychology of negotiating, in particular the results of psychometric testing. I came out as a very strong thruster-organiser and analyst and the psychologist wanted assurances that I had interests outside work. She was worried about my aggressiveness to achieve an aim. I reassured her I had a family and we all windsurfed together. I did not tell her about the family's competitiveness!

Anyway, BAE was obviously reassured and, once again, I gained this reputation for laying down policy. I saw the task as being like the production of the Blue Book[10] in the MOD and just as tome-like. Moving away from research made the job less interesting and Ros was first to leave, to work for the National Air Traffic System (NATS). As ever, she was quick to see the writing on the wall. I stayed but lost some interest.

The cost-cutting procedure was based on projects being numbered, to which workers booked, and if expertise was not required, booking was made to a waiting number. The longer people booked to the waiting number, the more vulnerable they became to redundancy. It was a neat system based on meritocracy but was extremely distressing to those in the margins and morale slumped. I was fireproof because I was an account holder and handed money to projects, but I felt the pressure. As time passed, more and more people

---

10 The Blue Book was the long-term plan for the RAF. The government and senior air officers did not like working to a long-term plan because it cut out the short-term options for financial and manpower changes.

were at my door, some in tears. I felt my job becoming more and more miserable. The Division's manpower reduced from 25,000 to eventually rest, once again, at 15,000. The redundancy payments, unlike in the steel and coal industries, were good and nothing seemed to leak into the newspapers.

Eventually, I felt so guilty and miserable at being one of the "hatchet men" that I evaluated my future and decided to stand on my own two feet: I formed my own company. After all, I now had a reputation for producing projects to time and budget.

My company was Research and Development Management Ltd (Radman).[11] So it was that I volunteered for redundancy after eight years at BAE and was handed a pension and a lump sum.

It was a smart move. The boys were growing up—Mark was off to university and John was working at a windsurfing shop and had met Kate, whom he would eventually marry—and Trish had a teacher's income. The time came when we didn't need the big house and we moved (yet again) to a small cottage on the edge of Gamlingay.

After forming my own company, I quickly settled into another company called Cambridge Associates with other consultants. I found my niche in mainly helping to design military war-gaming software. The

---

11 Radman was handed to my son-in-law, Chris, when I retired, and it was used to develop children's playgrounds.

company was called Flames, and I am quite sure the software was eventually declassified and must have been used in the gaming industry that was to start to grow in the 1990s. Again, the task was to provide analysts with conceptual advice about war at sea and in the air. It was very relaxing, for I was in control of the pace and type of my work. However, I saw myself as easing into retirement and I had time to enjoy the windsurfing with the family. I had also, at the age of fifty-one, become National Senior Champion of 1989. In many ways my cup was running over. My working life had been very exciting but somewhat stressful and, to be honest, I was beginning to feel the pace.

Chapter Five
The National Air Traffic Service

My plan to run slowly and peacefully into retirement was changed by one telephone call: it was from Ros. She had had a meteoric rise in the National Air Traffic System (NATS) and had become a director. She explained she had been at a recent board meeting discussing change and problems in NATS. At this stage NATS was still part of the civil service and they were having problems adapting to the market ethos thrust on them by the Thatcher government. The board was looking for a consultant to help them cope with change. Ros had declared she knew just the person they were looking for, hence the call. This was interesting because I had always believed that you should have time to talk to, and help, subordinates. I thought back to the time Oscar had called me, years after we had parted, and he had said he wanted to fly on my squadron again. Here again was a phone call from the past, but this time it was from an erstwhile subordinate who was now in a superior position. To say it inflated my ego was an understatement. I still trusted Ros's judgements, so accepted the challenge.

If I had known what was ahead, I might have been more circumspect because the road to retirement became bumpy.

The good thing was I remained independent, and NATS employed me as a member of Radman Ltd. I first thought there would be only one task and it would be relatively straightforward.

A new operations room for Airways and Initial Approach Control in the UK was being built at Swannick, the manning of which was causing concern. My job was to interview everyone in line for middle and higher management, to look at their capabilities, and to suggest how things should be managed in the future. It lasted a few interesting weeks, after which I submitted my report. As with the MOD, the civil servants were established for life (or so they thought) and they were comfortable with the way they managed things; they could see no reason to change. They gave me a strong message that they would fight to protect the culture as it was. Some thought the change had come too late in their careers and they would refuse to adapt. NATS was quite different from BAE, where change had been accepted with aggressive thoroughness. NATS was at the other end of the spectrum; inertia was the name of the game. I was also becoming aware of Masonic threads running through the organisation and binding it together. It was a bond I was quite unable to break.

Much to my surprise, I was told my report was of value, even though I felt little would change to meet the needs of Swannick. Indeed, problems *did* follow when Swannick was made operational.

I packed my bags to move on, but at the last moment I was asked to remain and take over a sister project that had run into difficulty. The project was known as the Central Control Function (CCF). It was an expensive and very important project that had been progressing slowly over time; now the last stage would not work.

CCF was a new operations room at Uxbridge. (Years later it was absorbed into Swannick.) The aim was to bring together, into one location, the approach control of all the major London airports, in order to allow free flow of traffic in and out of Heathrow, Gatwick and, most particularly, Stansted.

Thus, while Swannick was dealing with the upper airspace, CCF would control approaches to the runways. When I took over, much of the hardware to do with radar, computers and communication had been fitted. My task was to manage testing, operational release and the lead into manpower training. Above all, there was the task of changing the last phase.

The original concept of CCF was to take aircraft from the upper airspace and feed them into "tubes in the sky". These tubes would interlace from quite a long way out and allow aircraft an unfettered approach to one particular runway. It was a great idea that had been copied from the USA, but as the project progressed it was realised that it would not work. Unlike in the USA, there was a shortage of airspace available in the southern UK, principally due to it being so close to French and Netherland flight information regions (FIRs). So, software and training had to be re-engineered and reversed to go back to the stacking system but with the benefits of the co-location of approach control. Project packages were changed and I revised costs. As with the culture in the civil service, I found each level of management had added ten percent contingencies to the project. I handed back a six-figure sum. That put the cat amongst the pigeons! No one gave money back after commitments had been made about the need. I explained that performance, time and money had to be accurate. A balance was needed. Too much money could mean the project would relax and time would be extended. The money was "hidden" because no one could understand my way of thinking. However, the project was completed to time and my budget. Come the day of operational release, Princess Anne came to unveil a plaque. I stood my turn at the back of a queue to shake her hand and be congratulated. It was amazing how many people were involved with the management, and I had never seen them!

Eventually, the CCF coped with more traffic than it had been designed for, but it was some years before the function went to Swannick. Technology in the air has improved, but it is a matter of fact that the airspace over London is always a limiting factor. Extending the runway at Heathrow is more political than practical and Brexit was to shut off integrated development with airspace nearby. As I write, I wonder how runway extension will develop.[12] Why did we give Stansted the capacity to increase its business and then not let it develop? The hub to the UK is not just Heathrow; it is the whole group of London airports.

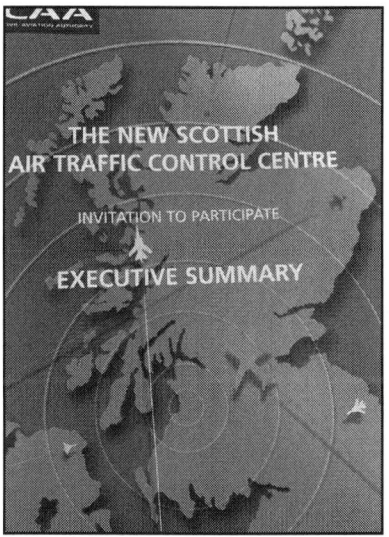

The cover of the brochure we produced as part of our work to get tenders to build the new air traffic control centre at Prestwick

---

12 Gatwick became favoured when more consideration was given to the problems of climate change.

With the success of CCF came another project and this could have been the biggest NATS project ever. It was to be run by a NATS director near the Civil Aviation Authority and NATS HQ in London. It was to be a totally new air traffic control centre at Prestwick and was so costly it was to be a private finance initiative (PFI) project. So back to London for me; I was to manage the production of the contract tender, or Invitation to Participate (ITP) as it was more politely put. It was not my cup of tea, but it was a good personal contract.

It was so very prescriptive that huge manuals were produced on requirements that covered everything in great detail, even down to how many millimetres the grass lawns had to be kept. We worked for a year, then—just when we were close to issuing the document—NATS itself was privatised. That was the end of the project. At that stage NATS had finished with my work because there were no more suitable problems for me to get my teeth into.

Earlier in the year, while I was working for NATS at Uxbridge and the whole family was getting well into windsurfing, I realised I was becoming stretched with the amount of time I was in the car during the week and at the weekends. In the back of my mind, I was thinking about the future. It was bad enough driving down the A1 and round the M25 twice a day, but every Friday I would arrive home and pack the car and a trailer full of windsurfing kit to head off with the family to a competition. It could be anywhere in the UK. Above all, I had just got completely fed up with the traffic on the M25. I decided that on some days during the week I would try to stop at Uxbridge, but what could I do? I remembered London and was not too impressed with the idea of another flat or B&B. Then I thought of the canal. What about a narrow boat?

Chapter Six
The Start of Our Travels

One day I took a break, walked down to the canal and found an office and club for the narrow boats. I really liked the set-up. I went back to the club and had a beer or two with people as they came and went. I enjoyed the facility, but when I looked more deeply into the ownership of a narrow boat, I realised it would take over my life and restrict family life. I sat in the clubhouse and pondered. After much deliberation, I proposed to buy a motorhome and park it at the clubhouse during the week. To my surprise, the family accepted the idea. They were equally surprised when I turned up with an Autotrail Chinook a few weeks later! I had paid £15,000. We named it Tardis because, once inside, it seemed to have a lot of space. However, it was not very good on the road and swayed badly in the wind and alongside large lorries. It was also very underpowered. Still, it did the job. I stayed in Tardis on Mondays, Tuesdays and Thursdays; Trish would sometimes visit during the week, and the motorhome was the source of family adventures at the weekend.

In time, the boys left home to lead their own lives,

but Trish and I could not break an old habit, and our life revolved around the motorhome and old windsurfers (the Seavets) in summer, and we went off to Spain from December to March.

One year, we had planned to leave on New Year's Eve, but storms were being forecast and so we changed plans and left early. We still hit the storms as we sailed to Saint-Malo and Trish was very apprehensive. However, she coped well with the crossing although there was no let up. All the way down south it blew and rained heavily, and Tardis wandered all over the road. Because it was winter, there were few places to stop, and we learned the need to plan in future for safety and security. The weather slowly improved and we meandered across Spain, enjoying the sights, to end up at Tarifa.

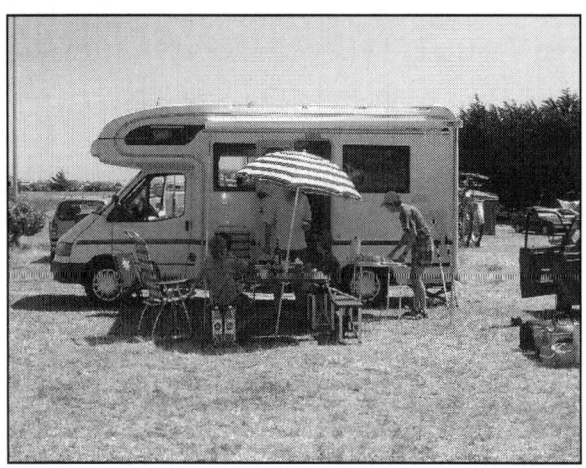

Trish and I preparing food for friends outside Tardis in Quiberon

On later trips we had a better motorhome. We bought it after forty-five years of marriage and it was called Ruby. It was powerful and pulled our laden trailer over the French and Spanish mountains effortlessly. We generally headed for Mercia, southern Spain, first. There we found a camping site right on the edge of the Mar Menor and alongside a military airbase. We settled there for the first half of the winter. Once the camp was struck, we rigged all our windsurfing kit and left it rigged up ready to windsurf when conditions were right. The conditions were benign, and Trish and I could sail together in safety. I had also learned that if we went on to Tarifa I needed to polish my windsurfing techniques and get physically fit. We made many friends while on the edge of the Mar Menor and each year the size of the parties increased. What pleased me most was to see how happy Trish was with our trips. But nothing stays the same forever and slowly there was a change in her mood, and she became more unsure about things.

Life was not all windsurfing. In December there were cold nights, and it was early days for the internet and digital TV, but we had a one-metre TV dish and, with a bit of luck and patience, we could get a signal from the UK. It could take a lot of fiddling. When I had it tuned in, others would look at us in the evening, wine in hand, watching Film4. They thought it was magic and I gained a reputation for setting up

TVs; that resulted in wine being deposited on our doorstep. What had made it easy for me was, wherever we stopped and set up the TV, I took a photo sighted down the receiver, then when back at the same location I would put a sighting device (a straight stick) on the object photographed. It was a simple extension of weapons development and operational assessment!

Usually, the first half of December was wet but gradually things improved; it got warmer day by day and was certainly much better than being back in the UK. Each year we met fellow windsurfers, ate well and drank wine. Once a week there was a practice air display by the Spanish "Red Arrows" from the airfield next door. During these pleasant and relaxing periods, I would run to get fit.

It was good to be settled and secure on a campsite because we had heard so much about seniors being attacked in their motorhomes, but it was just talk. That is, until it happened to us. We decided to travel by night and go sightseeing the following day. I had become tired while driving, so we paused under a light outside a café and went to sleep.

I woke up when I felt the cold night air on my face and wondered where the draught was coming from. As I pondered, I became aware of a hooded face dimly outlined above me. I was lying on my back and Trish was deeply asleep alongside me. I deduced that I was being watched, and the penny began to drop. I sat up quickly and shouted something very rude about the hooded head's parentage and hit out with a right hook that landed nowhere. He had expected my reaction and disappeared—with our precious bags—through the open door.

The next thought was, *Why the open door?* I soon found out my assailant had quietly cut out the quarter light, put his arm through and undone the lock. After collecting the glass, I went back into the motorhome, consoled Trish and realised passports, cash, credit cards and pills had gone; we were in a desperate situation, unable even to pay to get off the motorway.

I went outside to try to get a signal and ring the police, but no luck. Then I realised sitting on the ground were our two bags. I quickly checked inside. Lo and behold, there were our passports, pills and one of the credit cards. The cash had gone.

I was bemused and looked up to see the hood had a body, which was standing at a distance under a streetlight. It then waved on seeing my satisfaction at finding our bags. It was a case of *"adios, amigo"* and he was gone. I said goodbye to £60 and stopped the missing credit card. We travelled on. There was little point getting involved with the police.

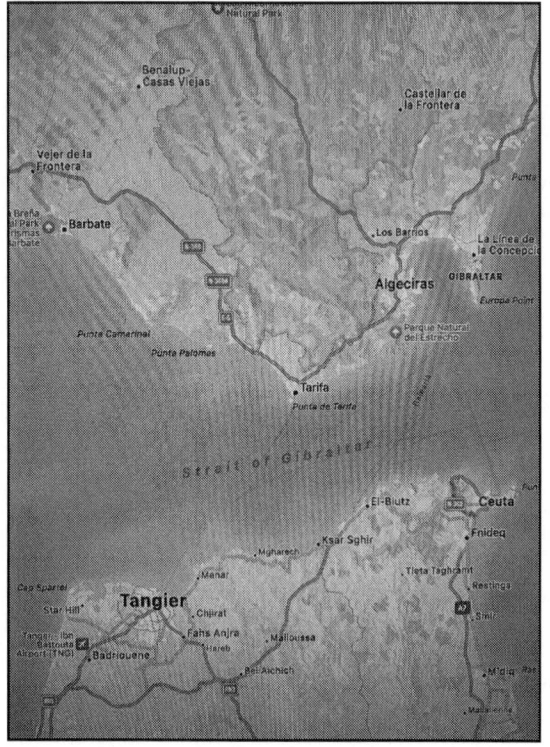

Map showing the position of Tarifa, where I learned to "dance the waves"

The plan, after stopping in the Mar Menor, was to head back carefully to Tarifa, which lies at the most southerly part of Europe and is the mecca of windsurfing. Across the Straits of Gibraltar can be seen the mountains in Morocco. The winds are either east or west and they are generally strong, kicking up magnificent waves around Tarifa. It is a challenge for even a young windsurfer, and I was sixty-four but up for the challenge. As I was to learn, I was the oldest there bar one. The other was a sixty-four-year-old Belgian who became my friend until he had a heart attack when struggling in the waves, but he came back about two years later after also suffering from prostate cancer.[13] He was made of the right stuff.

I so enjoyed my windsurfing at Tarifa! Sometimes, I would get way out close to Morocco and "dance" my way back on the waves. The scenery was beautiful and, as I "danced" and got closer to Tarifa, I could see the vultures soaring along the mountain tops. Vultures have such an ugly reputation but, on the wing, they are so graceful.

Back to Hurn. There was work for me. I was expected to refuse the offer, but instead I jumped at the idea. Not for the work, but the location was a mecca of windsurfing and Dorset would be great for retirement. It was a base from which we could head off windsurfing around Europe. It was now 1995 and I was fifty-eight years old.

---

13 Little did I know that I too would have heart problems, a cardiac arrest and prostate cancer some years later.

Chapter Seven
Retirement to Dorset and Dramatic Changes

It was up sticks again. Trish left her job at Sandy and gave up teaching. The family was left behind and we headed to the Poole area. We expected the children, now they were grown up, to go their own ways, but gradually over the months they headed to the South Coast. We always thought a London suburb was not a good place for our grandsons to be educated and grow up. Tina and Chris obviously started to feel the same way. There was a discussion about whether we should all live in the same house but, in the end, we decided we would move to the Wimborne area and Tina, Chris and the grandchildren, Maurice (Mo), Ciaran and Denzel, would move close by. Then the rest followed. John and Kate first moved to Southampton where John became a mature student and obtained a degree in Marine Science. When he finished, they also moved to Wimborne. Mark finished his degree in Film-making. For a while he worked in London, and then he and Bryony also moved to the Bournemouth area. Much later, Lesley finished her travels at sea and in Spain and then came to Wimborne, but there is a story to tell before this happened and Daniel, our oldest grandson, came to live with us. The final result was that the family members were to become close to one another again.

NATS had a building at Hurn Airport. On the top floor, at the corner of the building, I had an office overlooking the airfield. Most importantly, I could see the windsock and decide the wind strength and think about windsurfing. Every windsurfer has a tree or some such indicator of wind strength that is visible from a window. I had my own windsock. I could work at my desk and watch the aircraft and the wind. What a great start to a new job!

I was to manage software projects that NATS had won from the European Commission. Some were small, some were quite significant in the development of procedures to be used over the whole of Europe. It was at the stage of development of the internet that allowed people working on the projects, run by companies from across Europe, to work together without having face-to-face meetings. (Brexit was to change such cooperation.) We were breaking new ground in NATS by working on the internet, but there was extreme nervousness that we might pick up a virus and it would get into airport-control computers. We did get the occasional virus; red skulls appeared on our computers, and hooters sounded throughout the building. Panic would follow but it never actually amounted to much.

So, work pressed on from day to day and I would go home in the evenings. Of course, we did have meetings across Europe from time to time. If meetings were in Paris or Amsterdam, I could fly from Southampton in the morning and be home for tea having been hosted in an up-market restaurant for lunch. Sometimes it was in the south of France or Portugal and, exceptionally, I would be away for a couple of days. For two years until 1998, when I was sixty, it was a good life.

Trish was pleased as she had her own house and there was time for her to enjoy the grandchildren, who were eventually to grow in number to nine. She also enjoyed Seavets, a more mature organisation for windsurfers. She enjoyed their company for about a year alone, and when my competitiveness at UK events dwindled, I joined her.

The thought of living in happiness forever slowly changed. While we were living in our new home in Gamlingay, at the very start of our OAP adventures, I had a call from my Uncle Cyril saying he was ill and would like to meet up. I met him in hospital grounds at Rhyl while he was either waiting for a consultation or treatment. He told me he had prostate cancer, and the condition was terminal. He had waited six months for a diagnosis and, ironically, the consultant had said a diagnosis six months earlier would have given him a chance of survival.[14] We talked for a while and then he explained the problem of leaving Dolly (his wife and my aunt) behind. I was the last in his line. Dolly had one niece, Linda, but they had lost touch with her over the years. Then came the point of the visit: "Terry, when I am gone, would you please keep an eye on Dolly?"

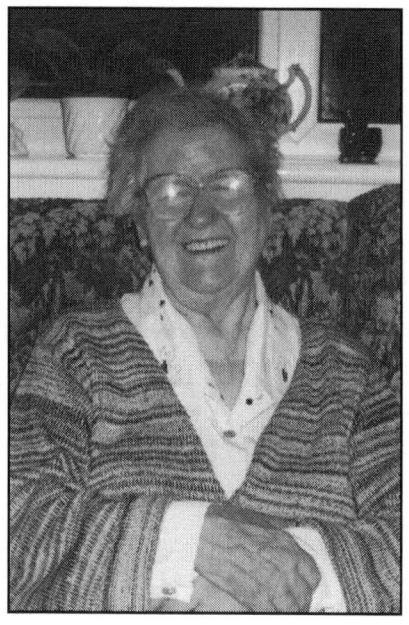

Aunt Dolly

Of course, I agreed to his request, and Cyril died a few months later.

---

14 As I write, there are considerable problems with the NHS. There have been good times but there have always been mistakes. It is the nature of the beast.

All seemed to go well for about two years. We would either visit Dolly and her three Scotties, or Trish or I would phone her, once a week. Then things seemed to go wrong. First, the conversations on the phone were a bit strange and then they became *very* strange.

Dolly had a very gentle nature and lived for her dogs. She had no friends we knew about and eventually, when contact virtually ceased, I rang her doctor and asked if he would be kind enough to call on her because we were worried about her condition. Well, as had happened with Cyril, she was very much abandoned. First, the doctor declined to help, so I jumped into my car on a Saturday morning and drove from Wimborne to Prestatyn.

When I arrived at her terraced house, I knocked on the door and the dogs barked. Then gentle Dolly started shouting like a mad woman saying all sorts of horrible things about how she was going to protect her house. I pushed open the letterbox to see what was happening in the house and the smell was awful! The dogs had obviously mucked everywhere, and they looked horribly thin. The doors and windows were firmly bolted and, short of bashing down a door, there was no way of getting in. I was concerned that, if I stayed there too long knocking and shouting, the neighbours might become offensive, so I left and visited the Social Services in Rhyl for advice or help.

Well, the reaction from them was about the same. It was Saturday and they had better things to do. They told me to go away and if I didn't stop bothering them, they would call the police.

I said that was a good idea, pulled up a chair and put it in the doorway to the manager's office.

"The police and an ambulance will be fine, and we can section my aunt and get her to hospital."

I sat there for about thirty minutes until the manager gave in. Sectioning would be arranged for mid-afternoon.

True to arrangement, an ambulance arrived with a policeman and a Social Services rep. This time it was the reverse. These officers simply folded their arms and told me to get on with it. The neighbours came out to watch the Saturday afternoon sport. I broke the lock on the front door and entered. The smell was beyond terrible, and I wanted to retch.

Dolly came to the doorway. Her hair was standing on end and her eyes were wild. I told her I wanted to look after her and she needed to go to hospital. I took her hand, but she was going nowhere. She then flew at her elderly, frail neighbour and I had to constrain her. She was so strong I was fearful my restraint was going to hurt her. At last, I received help from the ambulance crew.

Dolly went to hospital, and I was left looking at

three distraught dogs and a broken door. In late afternoon, the dogs were given shelter and the door was secured. I went to the hospital. Dolly was obviously sedated. It was explained that we had got her to hospital in time; she was suffering a critical stage of diabetes.

Of course, this was only the start of caring for her. She spent weeks in hospital recovering and there was no way she was ever going home. While she was in hospital, the first problem I needed to solve was what to do with the dogs. What I had arranged was very temporary, so I looked for a permanent home. I found a lady called Alma who cared for dogs. She and her blind husband lived in a very remote area where the Welsh mountains climbed skywards. Alma had an incredible reputation but, much as she loved looking after her dogs, she was strapped for time and cash. I offered an arrangement to help her income for the time the dogs survived. A deal was done, and we became friends.

That was just the start.

While Dolly was in hospital, I had to do something with the house, so back to Prestatyn. In came a professional house clearance firm and then came the cleaning. We realised her fight with diabetes had made her blind, so we decided to put Dolly in a home near us. *That* was easy enough to do, but it started a bureaucratic battle between councils, one in North

Wales and the other on the South Coast. I ended up with a file about two inches thick before financial arrangements were agreed. Unfortunately, the house was lying empty and I was forced to sell it at the bottom of the market by the Council. Nice little terraced house: £18,000 (just £3,000 more than we had paid for our motorhome). I was really fed up with the pressure put on me to get an instant sale.

However, it was a pleasure visiting Dolly. Despite losing her sight, she seemed contented, and members of the family supported me. Trish and I saw her from time to time. During our chats she told me of her friendship with Jean, my blood aunt and youngest sister to my father, Sam. I believe I wrote something about Jean in my earlier book. I said to Dolly, "Sam told me that Jean had died young of an embolism."

Dolly immediately replied, "Terry, that's just not true. There was an argument, and she was shot."

I was aware Dolly and Jean had been good friends. Their friendship had started when they worked together in an armaments factory during the Second World War and while Cyril was a prisoner of war. Because Dolly was not the sort of person to fib—and because she had been close to Jean—I believed her.[15]

---

[15] I have since looked through old papers and found that Jean had changed her name to Mrs Jean Ritchie. This reminded me of a discussion between my mother and father about Jean having met a black man. The 1950s… difficult in the past.

But I never went to Walsall to look for evidence.

Time went by and it was obvious diabetes had ravaged her body. While we were talking one evening, she became very weak and distant. I was holding her hand at the time and the conversation was waning.

"Dolly, you need some sleep."

"Yes, Terry. That's a good idea," she murmured.

I left her but was concerned, so I returned early in the morning to find she had died during the night. After a troubled life and the traumatic years, the ending was dignified and peaceful. She died about five years after moving south to be close to my family. We did the right thing by Cyril.

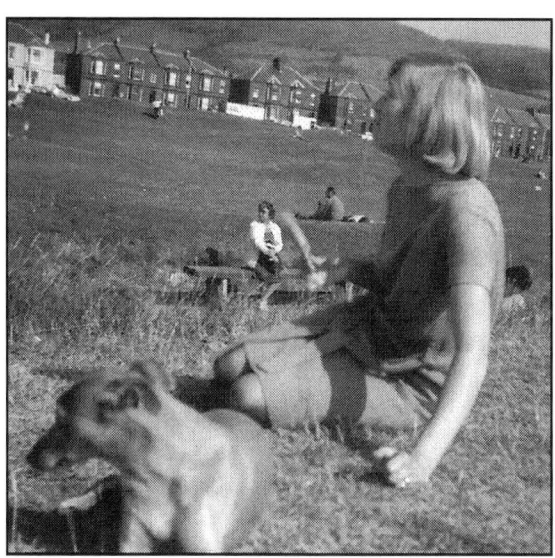

Trish's sister Phyllis, with Maurice's dog Muffet, in Scotland

Although my family roots were in Walsall, my mother, father, grandmother, Cyril and Dolly had all moved around. In their final years, my mother, father and grandmother lived together in a bungalow in Norfolk. When they died, they were cremated and their remains were placed under a rose bush in the gardens of the crematorium at Horsham St Faiths, near Norwich. I decided to take the ashes of Cyril and Dolly to rest there, with my family roots.

While we were struggling to care for Dolly, several things occurred that led me by the nose into retirement. In May 1997 there was a telephone call to tell Trish her younger sister, Phyllis, had a brain tumour and was in intensive care.

We went to see Phyl but she was in a coma from which she never returned. This shook Trish more than anything before, and she realised the last of her childhood family had gone. I had the same experience after my mother and Cyril's deaths. Trish's grief was particularly difficult for me to deal with. I didn't realise it at the time but this—and agricultural chemicals on farms and in Grafham Water—could have been the trigger for Parkinson's and my concern on our travels for Trish's change in demeanour.

At work, I got very angry with the French who were hijacking the engineering on a European project and trying to turn an airspace control project into a French national project. The project had gone through the conceptual and data-gathering stages run by the British and the Portuguese and everything had been agreed, as we began the engineering design to be run by the French. Problems came to a head at a Paris meeting hosted by Thomson-CSF. Thomson arranged coffee and lunch, which took up most of the day before members had to catch aircraft home. It became obvious they wanted minimum discussion and to let the meeting default to the French national project. I told them if they didn't do what had been agreed I would sack them and let another country take their place. No one did this to a European project and Thomson consulted board members before we left, and they promised to meet the previous agreement. But, as soon as we were all back home, it became obvious they were going to continue down a national road. The French were developing the habit of supporting European projects but only insofar as they could become French.

My headaches increased and I went to the doctor.

My professional life, as in the past, and the family illnesses and demises caused a very significant change in our lives. The doctor did not mince his words; he told me I had high blood pressure and—if I carried on pressuring myself—I would have a stroke and die.

He added that one of his patients, like me, had had a stroke while cycling up Rowlands Hill, Wimborne, and he had just been buried. I remembered his comment. Nearly twenty years later, Rowlands Hill was to become both my nemesis and my friend.

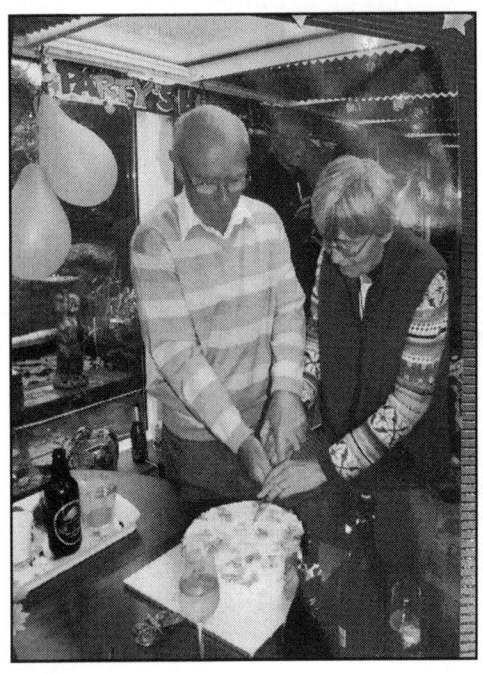

Golden Wedding Anniversary: Trish and I are cutting the cake

At this time Radman Ltd had been offered its biggest contract and I turned it down. So, at the age of sixty, I retired and turned to Trish and gave her priority and time for us to spend together. That time extended from 1998 to 2008 in time for our golden wedding anniversary. It turned out to be one of my better decisions, for we then had ten years totally in one another's company, travelling and free from other problems.

Still at work in 1996, and contemplating entry into retirement, we moved into a four-bedroom semi-detached house in Colehill, a mile from Wimborne. The location was chosen because it was close to the Canford Bottom junction, which would allow easy access east if I needed to go to London. It also put me on the road to Hurn, where I had my office and carried out my work for NATS and, most importantly, to the many windsurfing sites. There was an ample drive outside the house to accommodate motorhomes, trailers and cars. There was also a long tandem garage that took a large inventory of windsurfing kit with room for a large sewing machine to make windsurfing sails. It was all quite idyllic. We did not see any clouds on the horizon.

Chapter Eight
The Future and a Glance Back

For the next part of my story, I will jump forward eighteen years, or so, for a break in my story and to reminisce about my past at the time of retirement.

One early morning, I lay on my back and looked at the ceiling of a flat. I was no longer in the house or the bungalow I had bought to please Trish. I was conscious of a shaft of sunlight entering the bedroom. It was my habit to lie there and think, not that I had had a sleepless night—for I always went to bed and slept deeply—but the early morning was when I organised my day and thought about life and the universe. Some thinking was good, but to ponder too long was not good because troublesome thoughts could start the day badly. On this particular day, I was just lying there and wondering how I had arrived at this point in life. I was seventy-six for Christ's sake and had been retired for sixteen years; why didn't I just sit in a rocking chair and rock peacefully? Surely that was what was expected of me?

But I lay there. It was to become a long and thoughtful lie-in as I realised just how accidental the path through life was. True, I had been very focused on my career even when I was a teenager. I wanted to fly, and nothing was going to stop me. I even cheated in medical exams to achieve this aim. I asked myself the question: "Why - if you can work and cheat to meet the aims of a career - are love, family life and health all so accidental?" And why, in my case, have work and married life been so continuous, while others have fallen at every fence and never seemed able to pick themselves up? It was not that I was anything special with regard to intellect or physique. So, what was the answer?

I thought long and hard that morning and concluded that there were two aspects to my life. One was totally out of my control, in that I was lucky. Hence the expression "luck is my shadow", the title of my book about my early years. The second was in my character; I had been very opportunistic. If I had seen opportunities, I grabbed them. Yes, I never waited patiently for the best. I would just grasp the good and it was a matter of luck that things turned out for the best. Unfortunately, with age, opportunities seem to fade with the lucky shadow that went with them.

I jumped out of bed and started my day. It had been a good thoughtful start, and I would return to try to answer how I had arrived at old age without quite understanding the latter part of the journey. How was it that I had come to lie in bed in a flat in a gracious house in Dorset on this particular morning? I dressed, gave my new wife a peck on the cheek, tucked her in as she slept, and crept off to Costa to have a quick coffee and to read *The Times*.[16]

Mary, at the age of sixty-six, was disabled with Parkinson's disease, yet it was she who slept so peacefully. I had travelled through life on a path full of problems and adventures with twists and turns that had mainly been made by accident or by the hands of others. Yet, here were Terry and Mary, newlywed, in love, and quite bemused at their luck in finding one another. The stories of Romeo and Juliet were not always about youth and unhappy endings. However, it was late in life and love is different. For in place of passion is the need for love, understanding and especially tolerance. Once again, I headed off, confident of the journey ahead. Little did I know how things could change.

---

16 My quick coffee (over an hour) was repeated almost daily for more than fifteen years. I would write another book. I met and made so many friends I was to call them "my other family". In the depressions of old age and poor health they stopped me from going mad.

Chapter Nine
Parkinson's

I never really understood how Parkinson's entered my life, for it was present as early as 1979. It was like a child tugging at my trouser leg while I was busy having an adult conversation. I tried to concentrate on "the conversation" but Parkinson's, like the child, was determined to get my attention.

Trish's father, Maurice, was first to get Parkinson's and was the "child" looking for attention. Maurice had three children: Rex was the eldest, then there was Trish (originally called Pat), and the youngest was Phyllis. Life was complicated for all of us, and we had little time and understanding for this difficult newcomer. I look back at the situation with great regret, nay even guilt, but it was the start of my education in what was to follow, and slowly the seeds of understanding developed.

Maurice lived in the Forest of Dean. His wife, Molly, had died the decade before this difficult child arrived. His real children were scattered, and his friends and neighbours were infirm or dying; such is the problem of old age. The rest of us were in the middle of our careers, busy, self-indulgent and not caring enough to truly understand the problem he was carrying and that was weighing him down. Research now has shown that Parkinson's starts a decade or so before symptoms show themselves. I am not sure how it started for Maurice. He was always a bit introspective, but things must have been gathering in his mind before he went to the doctor's. When he was told he had Parkinson's disease, I am not sure he really understood what was happening to him. For the rest of us, he just focused on two things: television and food. He was certainly not a difficult man to look after. The doctor informed him there was a place for him in a care home, but he became ashamed of this news and told no one. In any case, the children would have encouraged him to go into the home and they could have got on with their complicated lives. It is always the easy way out for a busy family.

To be fair to Maurice's children, it was more than just complicated. One by one they were going into crisis.

Rex, the eldest, was married to an alcoholic and his days were a nightmare. The drinking eventually killed his wife Clare. After her death, he married a nurse with two children. Then he got cancer and died. In fairness, Rex was overwhelmed by his problems.

Phyl, the youngest, lived miles away in Scotland. There was the problem of the long distance from the Forest of Dean. And was Phyl aware of what was happening to her and her brain?

Trish also had her own problems, to which was added the problem of living with the complexity of my life in the Falklands and Cold Wars, and time away running a board of inquiry and a fighter squadron.

Not knowing, or asking, about care homes, the children decided to "share" Maurice. So it was that Maurice travelled between his children's homes in Scotland, Wales and Lincolnshire. Now anyone who knows anything about Parkinson's knows there is a search for a routine, friendly support and reassurance. Unfortunately, Maurice's family circumstances mitigated against these requirements. I felt uncomfortable, but I too was guilty of shrugging my shoulders and immersing myself in my own problems. Later, I was in a position to watch this situation repeat itself over and over again in other families.

Parkinson's is not in itself a fatal disease, so it is said, but it wears the individual down and in Maurice's case allowed angina to develop and for heart disease to leave him defenceless. It is a bit like foot soldiers wearing an army down to the point that the cavalry can sweep through and carry out the *coup de grâce*. The immune system can weaken, and a fall or minor infection becomes a major threat.

Maurice was gone and the family problems at the time of Maurice's illness were also history. Rex and Phyl had gone too. Trish and I were lucky to reap some of the benefits of a slightly early retirement. We could at last be together after a lifetime of struggle with jobs, separation and child-rearing. We were enjoying travel in a motorhome, playing golf and windsurfing. Then it happened.

Trish was a really good windsurfer and for her age she was quite exceptional. Then she started falling off her board and, more and more, I was recovering her and bringing her home. Then she became unsteady on her bike and her gait became reminiscent of her father's. We were walking along a country path in Spain, and I said, "Is it time we spoke to a doctor?"

Trish then became very angry for she knew I had opened up a discussion that was at the back of both of our minds.

"You think I have Parkinson's?" She spat the words out, but we both knew we could be in denial no longer.

We came back to the UK and went to the Parkinson's consultant; it took him only a few minutes to agree with our own assessment. We were about to enter Maurice's world that we had treated so casually, the difference being it was much closer to home for both of us. The "tugging child" now had my full attention, and I was about to enter the world of old age, infirmity and the limitations of the NHS and care in general.

It is a great shock to learn your nearest and dearest has been diagnosed with an awful disease, even if you are expecting it. The next day you feel life has changed completely and utterly. Perhaps it has, but most of the change is in your head. The real change is going to be a slow and cruel grind, and it is the grind that almost all disabled must deal with.

After the initial shock is a period of disbelief. In Trish's case we decided to test things and went on a package holiday to Minorca for Trish to see if her windsurfing was finished. But in supported conditions, while she could do some windsurfing, there was a real problem. It actually *was* the end of windsurfing and the end of cycling. Never mind! There was still the motorhome for travel and sociability. We would just have to adapt and cope with the grind.

The diagnosis took place early in the new millennium and I started to consider, as ever, where we stood regarding luck. I considered the adage that there was always someone else who was far worse off, which is true, but what happens to you is so real and personal. My doctor had shaken my complacency about an impending stroke, and I retired from work. There followed two years during which we would entirely devote time to one another. By the year 2000 there was the consolation that, unknowingly, I had done the right thing. We had been close to one another daily for two to three years, something which had been difficult to achieve over the previous fifty-plus years.

Chapter Ten
Caring and Old Age

The next few years passed with only slow change. There was an increase in the type and number of drugs taken by Trish, but we held back from taking dopamine drugs in the form of Madopar and Sinemet until about 2005 because of the warning that they were useful for only a limited amount of time. Nevertheless, mobility was decreasing and, worst of all, there was a mental change when everyday procedures became difficult to remember.

Trish started to take Sinemet, and the reducing mobility stabilised, but hallucinations began to set in, and memory of day-to-day routines started to fail. Dementia with Lewy bodies was the new problem to be understood. While this form of dementia did not appear to be as aggressive as Alzheimer's, I learnt its prognosis was not good. We were beginning to face real, intrusive problems from which there was little relief. The job of caring became a twenty-four-seven job, and I felt the pressure. In addition, Trish's mobility was erratic. I felt I could cope but I started to think about the future. During this early period, we were still able to travel and on some days I would find the old Trish, but I had complicated life by also looking after Daniel, our eldest grandson, who had broken his leg badly in Spain. I had brought him home to England to recover and to get him into an English school.

Thus, my caring responsibilities increased and the tasks of taking a young teenager to footballing activities and to school started to fill my days. To begin with, all was well. Daniel had time to learn to play golf and was also a good golfing companion to me. But things were going downhill for his mother and brother in Spain.

Lesley had sold her house after her divorce, bought a boat with the proceeds, and headed off with a new partner. The whole situation troubled Trish and me and we worried about our other grandson, Charlie, on a boat in Spain trying to get some sort of education in a foreign language. I would have liked to bring Charlie home too, but I knew I would not cope. In fact, I saw Bob Mitchell, the partner, enjoying that situation and he would have taken Lesley into all sorts of trouble without any of her children. I just did not trust him, but he *was* Lesley's partner, and I did not want to offend her by speaking my mind. However, in hindsight I should have taken a stronger stance because when Bob fell out with Lesley, he became violent and hurt her, then stole the boat and disappeared. Lesley returned home to Dorset with Charlie, broke and distressed. Some of the distress was shared by the rest of the family.

Daniel was growing up and we shared an anger about Bob's actions. Goodness knows what would have happened if we had found him! We all spent weeks trying to find the boat. It was eventually found in dry dock in Portugal. Bob had run out of money and abandoned the boat. Eventually, Lesley and her two sons were reunited in Colehill, not far from the rest of the family. She started to put her life back together. She was also helpful to me, and Trish could see more of her daughter. For me, there was the realisation I had to organise for the future.

I decided to give up our four-bedroom house for a bungalow. Once again, the timing was significant because John, our elder son, needed more space for his business. He was uncertain about taking on another house and mortgage and would have liked to let his house and to rent family accommodation, but in the end, for the sake of family stability, he took our house and we moved into a bungalow at the bottom of Colehill, near Wimborne. Trish was delighted with the move because it had a beautiful, well-established garden. I was uncertain because I knew I was going to have to become a gardener as well as a carer, but when her face lit up and she saw the garden with its trees and fish ponds I knew it had to be our new home. If I had known the work I was going to have to do to look after trees, bushes and fishes, I might not have been so accepting.

We settled into the bungalow and had a great get-together for our golden wedding anniversary. For a time, it all seemed idyllic but then Trish's hallucinations and memory got worse. Her mobility also got worse, and Trish found it very difficult to climb up the motorhome steps. Once inside the motorhome, showering and cooking became difficult. It was also difficult to move the motorhome for shopping, and my time was totally consumed with chores. So, the motorhome went, and I bought a caravan.

I was aware that that this would be for a limited time too, but it was easy to shower and cook and move Trish around. We took the caravan to Quiberon, in northern France, and I realised that even this mode of living was limited. The hallucinations became dominant, and I spent a lot of my time "fighting commandos and wild animals", but we were amongst Seavets, and they were good company. This was our last travel adventure together. We came home, the caravan went and we retired to life in the bungalow. If I thought I had had stressful and testing times in my life, the next few years were to crown them all.

It soon became obvious it was going to be really difficult to move Trish, and just as difficult for me to get out and shop and do anything for myself. I took advice from Social Services. They offered some "sitting" long enough for me to do some shopping.

I could also save up time long enough to play nine holes of golf. During the day I had to watch Trish like a hawk. She had sufficient mobility to make tea and try to cook, but it was not easy. Tea could consist of five cups for the two of us with ingredients in separate cups and we could have milky water, or scalding water on its own, or a teabag in cold water.

We ended up with a couple of dangerous situations. The first was when the electric kettle was put on the gas ring, but luckily I was back in the kitchen in time to put out the fire. The next was one evening after I had fed her, was dog-tired and dozed off alongside her. She switched the gas on and left it. After that, I switched the gas off at the mains to the oven and only switched it on again when I tried to cook. Getting respite became more and more difficult but I found that, like clockwork, Trish would sleep from about 5 to 9 a.m. and I used this time to slip out to Costa and get a coffee and croissant. And that is how the long-lasting habit continued.

Of course, the family tried to help, but work and school schedules were demanding. It was at this time that Lesley moved back into rented accommodation and Daniel went home. Lesley found time to look after Trish and to let me play golf, but my health was inevitably sliding. I was not exercising properly, although I found some time for yoga, and I was eating anything that came to hand. Looking back, this was the start of a period that was to damage my health permanently, and my mental health was not in great shape either.

Trish had a habit at this stage of emptying drawers and scattering the contents. It was not a big deal, just another stressful situation on top of everything else, especially if I was to wake up at 2 a.m. and find Trish on the rampage.

One night it came to a head. I got out of bed to console her and found I could not move; my feet were frozen to the floor. I tried to talk to her, but she did not understand, and I panicked. I went to the doctor and said I needed help to cope. I was given some rotten pills with awful side effects. I gave them back to him and said I was not going down that route; I would rely on exercise and yoga. I went out and bought an exercise bike. It was a good decision, but it did not solve all the problems because Trish was almost beyond my control.

Chapter Eleven
A Horrible Decision

At this stage we started to use a wheelchair. Lesley and Trish's friend Geraldine were able to take her out for coffee from time to time, but even this became problematic. I could see Lesley hadn't come home from domestic problems in Spain to be immersed in domestic problems in Dorset.

I was slow, but it finally clicked that perhaps I was not just trying to deal with a wife with Parkinson's. Something else was going on. I spoke to her doctor, but the doctor did not understand, and it was decided that I should speak to a geriatric consultant. The consultant was kind and Trish answered his questions, then he analysed the situation. I was impressed at his care. He summed up the situation thus: "Your wife is allergic to the Sinemet. I have seen this situation before."

I asked, "So, what do we do?"

The consultant replied, "I am afraid there is no easy answer, but we have a choice." (What he really meant was: "You, Terry, must decide.") "We can reduce the dopamine and her mind will clear, but she will become totally immobile."

I just looked at Trish and said, "I want you back."

She knew what I was talking about. It was a horrible decision to make, but it was the right decision: the drugs were to be reduced. It was to take a period of weeks to carry out the reduction. What I did not understand was how the effects of immobility would take place, and seeking advice and understanding in the NHS was going to be an awful process.

I started the reduction and the hallucinations started to disappear, but she could no longer get out of the chair. I had to provide support for her to walk and the wheelchair gradually became a *must*. Then the conversations returned and then came my wife of old. I could provide better care for her and the stress on me reduced. But just when I thought things were better balanced, she became ill and I became very concerned.

With hindsight, it might have been that the drugs had been withdrawn too quickly, but something had happened. I rang the doctor and explained that Trish was lying virtually unconscious.

Chapter Twelve
The NHS Has Problems

The doctor arranged for a bed in hospital, and I agreed I would get her there. A bed was allocated in the geriatric ward. As we started the journey Trish wasn't too bad, apart from being distressed. When we arrived at the hospital, I went to Reception and was told the bed was not ready and we would have to go to A&E and wait. It was 10 a.m. and it was Good Friday 2009. At first, there were two or three people sitting around waiting, but soon the waiting room became crowded. A young nurse took Trish's temperature and blood pressure, and we waited. The electronic noticeboard initially showed a one-hour wait, then two, and it steadily increased to seven hours.

As time went by, the room became stuffy, and it was difficult to get water and food. Trish became upset and we became the centre of attention in the crowded conditions. The truth of the matter was that senior doctors, consultants and nurses had gone on Easter holiday. There was only a skeleton staff in the hospital, and there was little experience and expertise. It was Friday evening before the bed was made ready and Trish was taken to the geriatric ward. She had some food and drink but there was no one available to get her to the toilet except me. It was late evening when she was settled in bed. It had been a hell of a day. Trish went to sleep, and I went home to get some rest. It was obvious I was going to be needed early in the morning and I was certainly not going to be limited by visiting-hour restrictions.

I went in early the next day and made my way to Trish's bedside. It was quiet, oh so quiet! Bodies were lying in beds and there was a young nurse on duty.

"Has Trish seen a doctor?" I asked.

"No," she replied, adding, "The doctor in charge of the ward will be back Tuesday."

I challenged, "But what happens if there is a crisis?"

"There is a registrar in A&E."

"We were in A&E yesterday and there was a seven-hour wait. You must be joking," I retorted.[17]

It was actually no joke. Neither was the situation in the ward. The nurse was obviously young and inexperienced, and for the next three days I was constantly by Trish's side to ensure she was fed and to take her to the toilet. Something else was happening: her head was dropping and it was becoming more

---
17 For me this was the birth of many of the NHS problems which were to become endemic by 2024.

and more difficult to raise it. Of course, there was no one with whom I could discuss the matter. Shoulders were shrugged. Knowing what I know now, I should have created merry hell and insisted on a neck brace being fitted, but I was also learning by experience and making mistakes.

Roused by Trish's situation, I put my management consultant hat on from the past. When Trish was asleep, I decided to tour the hospital and look at facilities and other wards. I started my tour, and it was quite obvious no one was going to intervene. I was right to think the place was lacking in manpower and there was lack of experience at all levels. It appeared to me that the higher the pay, the more likely it was that individuals had gone away to enjoy the rewards of their qualifications and the hospital was left to manage as best it could. I was sure individuals would swear that their vocational urge was there as ever but, although the NHS may have had some centres of excellence, organisational ability was at an abysmal level. I continued my tour. I passed expensive capital equipment, outpatient departments and laboratories quite devoid of activity. Applying some very simple calculations made me think that this huge building was only fully working 70% of the time.

I then thought back to my time in the RAF and, in particular, to flying squadrons during the Cold War. My thoughts also dwelled on those military personnel in Iraq and Afghanistan. Manpower was exceedingly short, yet still they had to cover tasks 24/7. I, personally, had had to show leadership by sharing duties over Christmas, Easter and weekends. It was a matter of honour that the lowest in rank had time off and the highest in rank shared the burden and provided an organisation that was resilient in working day and night. There was also high personal risk; even in the Cold War, I had lost my closest friends.

Fighting health issues is also a war fought every day of the week. I started to feel anger at an organisation that kept the lowest paid holding the fort while the highest rank and highest paid deserted the ship. I was starting to learn a lesson: not to trust those who were entrusted with my family's survival. Nothing was going to be taken for granted in the future.[18]

I struggled through to Tuesday morning and waited for doctors, senior nurses and physios to turn up and, of course, the inevitable happened. Problems had accrued over the weekend and the day was spent finding out what had happened while they were away and then prioritising issues that had built up while expertise was elsewhere. A doctor visited the ward but was short of time. He did not understand Parkinson's and just recorded that Trish was poorly. Later, I was

---

18 This thought was to lie heavily on my mind as the years passed. My trust in the Conservative Government's ability, and even in the NHS, faded. As I got older, I kept reminding myself that the buck stopped with me.

told I no longer had the capability to look after Trish and she should go into a nursing home. There was a hint she was dying, although it was not put into words. I told the doctor it was not for us to decide whether Trish should go into a home; I would speak to her and ask her opinion.

I spoke candidly to Trish, and she replied, "Terry, I see the sense of going into a nursing home, but I am losing the will to fight anymore. You will have to fight for me."

Those words burnt into the fabric of my being and, together with what I had seen on that fateful weekend, put me on a mission. I was damned if I was ever going to be pushed around again by a disorganised bureaucracy. (If only this had been true. In the years to follow, I was to be sucked into chaos again and again.)

Over the next week or two it became obvious that Trish's head would not rise again. She had dropped-head syndrome which was to stop her speech, starve her, and ulcerate her chest. The fight was obviously going to be exceedingly difficult.

The next surprise was when I was summoned to a meeting. I entered a small room where, seated round a table, were a social worker, the doctor and a nurse. The social worker led the discussion.

"We understand that Mrs Adcock has consented

to go into a nursing home, and we have allocated a place in Christchurch."

I was horrified. There was a pregnant pause while I thought out how to handle the situation. Christchurch was miles away. How could I look after Trish at such a distance? I would wear myself out on the road. I was even thinking this was meant to keep us apart. I gathered my thoughts, stood up with folded arms (in order to give myself maximum ascendancy) and said firmly, "To accept such an offer would be over my dead body. It is far—too far—away. *I* will choose the location and let you know my decision."

Chapter Thirteen
Trish Goes Into a Home

There was a stunned silence while they just stared at me and let it sink in that I had not only stood up but was resolute. They then tried to pressure me by saying I would have just twenty-four hours to make my decision.

The next day I visited care homes that were local to me, and I soon focused on a care centre which was just three miles away. I was particularly impressed by the caring attitude of the manager and her deputy, who were both very experienced nurses. It was not possible to get close to the rest of the staff, but those I met were kind to me. The home was set in very peaceful grounds and the whole place looked clean and organised. It was naughty that I had been given such a tight deadline in the meeting the day before, especially as we were bound to be a paying client and would have to give up Trish's pension.

The centre responded quickly and assessed Trish in hospital. The deal was done within the twenty-four hours. Trish moved into the home soon afterwards, and no doubt the hospital was pleased to have a bed back and to recover from the Easter debacle. I was given access to the home any time day and night. It seemed we had made the very best of a stressful situation. However, the seriousness of dropped-head syndrome was beginning to sink in. Also, the manager and her deputy, who had impressed me so much, had their own plans. They were so good they were off to set up a care home of their own and Trish's home was about to go into a period of turbulence which lasted throughout Trish's time there.

The manager and the deputy left. There may have been other reasons for their departure that were not visible to me for, after they left, experienced carers also left, and managers came and went. Any continuity of care went with them. The manpower level became inadequate and, when one of the managers tried to correct things, it was obvious she was out of step with company headquarters. In my opinion, a financial squeeze was taking place and their duty of care was getting lost. I wasn't worried for Trish, as I had promised to fight for her. I started to make decisions and take more and more of the burden of care onto my own shoulders. This was bound, eventually, to put me at odds with the changing management and company headquarters, but I had my own mission and, if they were going to fail with theirs, mine was going to be met.

After six months or so, the difference between the

system and me increased. I started to fight on three fronts. The first was a clash with the Council and NHS about funding; the second was the continuing disagreement about care and staff in the home; and the third was a great difference of opinion with the visiting doctor about Trish's right to survive.

Looking back, I realise the three-year period while Trish was in the care home put a pressure on me that would be a drag on my health. My windsurfing was dwindling to a close, but I did some yoga whenever possible and there was a spare space on a mat. I played nine holes of golf when I could, and very occasionally managed eighteen holes if the family went in or trusted carers were on duty. But the mental pressure was great. I ate what was available rather than being sensible, in contrast to years past. Costa opened early in the morning, so it was easy to break my journey with a coffee and I was beginning to meet and get to know people in Wimborne who were quite separate from my problems.[19] At night the easy option was a snack in a nearby pub.

I bought a Skoda diesel, but I could not take it on long journeys to clear the filter, so in the end had to change it for a petrol version. My journey from the bungalow to the care home was three miles and, on

---

19   I continued to go to Costa very early in the day for the next fourteen years and continue to do so. I have made friends with a lot of people whom I now call "my other family".

average, I did the double journey three times a day. I would break the journey to shop for Trish and go home to rest when she was asleep. I drove 30,000 miles driving backwards and forwards during Trish's time in the home. I became "invisible" to a lot of my past friends, and I ignored a certain tiredness, which I eventually accepted might have been the start of a heart problem. Some friends and family found it difficult to visit Trish and, in many ways, we became a fortress on a lonely island, but then we held this old-fashioned view about love and marriage.

Chapter Fourteen
Care and Finance

Almost as soon as Trish was settled in the care home in 2009, there was a message that a financial assessor would like to meet me at my home to discuss our financial contribution. We met as requested and questions about Trish's funding were put to me, for I had Power of Attorney. As we delved down into the detail, I said I would have to switch on the computer to see a spreadsheet about the details of Trish's pension. I answered all the questions, and it became obvious that I would have to hand over her pension and make contributions of Trish's cash until it had reduced to a basic level. The good thing was the bungalow was in joint ownership and, as I was living in it, that could not be touched.

The assessor then had the cheek to ask me about my income and wealth; I told her that was none of her business and she backed off. Then I told her that, while I was in general agreement with her assessment (I had read the regulations), Trish, as part-owner of the bungalow, still had some responsibility for its upkeep and some of her pension should be allocated for that purpose. She immediately agreed, although she had not mentioned this before. What a cheek! And what a hidden threat to others!

Of course, the home was expensive, and it didn't take many months for Trish's finances to reduce to the minimum. At that stage I decided to try to move the responsibility from the Council to the NHS by claiming Continuing Healthcare. The deputy and head nurse at the home received a "machine code" document to complete. It was a complicated document, and it took hours to complete. Although Trish was bed-ridden, the claim failed. In truth, the claims nearly always fail; there is not the money to support such a system.

However, Continuing Healthcare support existed, so I had another go. This time *I* filled in the application and inserted photos into the document. There were no threats, but this could be seen as a document that the media would understand. The claim was one of the few accepted in Dorset. I felt guilty that I had achieved what other deserving cases had not. Thinking back to Easter, I consoled myself that others at the highest level in the NHS were taking as much money and time as they could get. In some ways it was a dog-eat-dog situation with regard to NHS funds. Years later, poor government, a pandemic, isolation from Europe, inflation and greedy strikes took things to a low level that I thought was hardly possible to achieve.

The problems in the care home waxed and waned. Sometimes care would get better and sometimes it was awful. Inevitably, standards went downhill, and the shortage of staff (especially experienced staff) was an ever-increasing problem. I could have moved Trish to another home, but in the end, I decided I would accept the care home's capabilities and make up the difference myself. I just did not want to risk the frying-pan-and-fire syndrome.

Thus, Trish was protected, but when I had time to think of others, I felt so sad. I watched families dump their elderly then go away and argue about money, never to be seen again. In the depths of winter—when the infections arrived—the doctor would visit, rooms would empty and black bags would be discreetly taken away by smart vans with "Private Ambulance" written over the windscreen. The elderly would die with no one there to hold their hands. They would just be discovered cold at breakfast time. Of course, there were some really caring relatives, but I am sad to say they were few and far between. I was beginning to understand that our culture allowed us to talk about care while not being excessively involved with it. Certainly, I was as guilty as most when I looked back to my working years.

Chapter Fifteen
Care Becomes Dangerous

Unfortunately—although I thought Trish was protected—it was not quite true, and I became aware of my limitations quite early on. I had visited Trish at breakfast time one day. She was fed and washed and went to sleep. As usual, I saw this as the time I could go to the shops and have a haircut. I returned just before lunch and entered her room. The bed was empty. I turned to the chair, but she was not there, or so it seemed. Where was she? No one would have taken her out in a wheelchair because I usually did that.

Then I looked at the chair again.

Oh no! There was a slipper and a leg sticking out from the back of the chair. I went quite cold.

One of the carers had lifted her out of bed and put her in a chair with an extra squab underneath her in such a way that the arms of the chair could not retain her. She had wanted the toilet, but no one had come, so she had squirmed her way over the sunken arm. She had then rolled backwards and was wedged upside down behind the chair.

I yelled for help and my voice boomed throughout the home. I pulled Trish out onto the floor and into the recovery position. She was very cold, and her mouth and nose were absolutely full of mucus. I thought she was drowning in her own fluids. I hooked out her tongue and cleared her nose and throat. I then cuddled her in blankets and talked to her. Her eyes flickered and she was back with me.

I was then conscious that the nurse had arrived. She just looked at the situation and froze. She did nothing because she was so frightened of the consequences; such was the fear between management and staff. I then found a carer and a hoist, and we got Trish back into bed. I had a one-way discussion with the manager about care and visits to rooms. It did not have much effect and my trust reduced even further. I was to spend even more time with Trish and my notes to management increased. The following is the text of a note to the manager, and it certainly was not isolated:

> *I just knew there were going to be problems this morning. It was 8.15 when I arrived. I saw Trish and quickly established that she needed to drink. She also needed the toilet, and her neck was bleeding quite badly.*
>
> *I looked at the situation with all the nursing tasks in hand and said I would feed Trish, but I would need help in about half an hour with the other problems.*

At about 9.15 I realised that the carers and nurses were still occupied, and I cannot blame them for they were working hard to meet their other duties.

By 10.15 I had fed Trish as best as I could, but her neck was hurting, and she did not want to use the pad; the discomfort in trying to keep dry stopped her from eating. I put her on the commode, changed the pad, washed her, changed the bed, stopped the bleeding, made Trish comfortable and cleaned the room. I had spoken to the carers, but the nurse had been the only one to visit room 11 (with the dopamine).

I left in a bad mood, but with the promise that Trish's neck would be looked at when there was time and in the hope that her top would be changed. It hasn't helped that the pictures of the wound have been lost (they were meant to be sent to another hospital) and their loss has not been rectified. From noting that there is a need for another nurse to be involved it will now take some weeks just in the notification stage.

I cannot help how I feel but I am now very, very angry.

The sore on the neck caused by the dropped-head syndrome and its effect on eating were causing Trish's weight to fall away. As the weeks passed, she became unable to talk to me. I decided something had to be done and this led to an argument with the visiting doctor. At this stage I was surprised the doctor could not see some of the problems in the home, but later I became aware that the power of a big company with its legal staff was frightening to those employed by the company and even to relatives and those in the caring profession.

Trish's weight dropped from sixty-two kilograms to an eventual thirty-two kilograms. She was so light that it was easy for me to carry her like a baby, and it was also kinder because it did not hurt her like the transfer to and from hoists. It was against the rules for me to pick her up, but I could quickly get her into a wheelchair and take her into the garden, or into the lounge, and feed her. In fact, it was to lead me to another impulsive decision. Trish told me how she had really enjoyed our travels in the motorhome and said how wonderful it would be to see the sea again. So, I spent my pension on a small motorhome that had good access and swivelling seats.[20] I was then able to carry her, or get our son John to help me carry her, to the motorhome. She would lie strapped in the reversed front seat, and I could make her tea and feed her, and she could look out to sea. But it was a difficult day out for me, and toilet requirements were very difficult. Throughout it all, eating and deteriorating communication were by far the most difficult problems and my deafness did not help.

---

20 It was the small motorhome which was to become my own home later when things became really difficult.

Chapter Sixteen
A Doctor Makes Me Very Angry

In a pensive mood, I had put Trish in the wheelchair and was taking her into the lounge when I saw that the doctor was visiting. I stopped to speak to her and said, "I have been giving the head drop some thought and I am sure there is a way of releasing the jaw so my wife can eat better."

I think I caught the doctor on a bad day because she replied, "Why don't you just accept things as they are and let her go?"[21]

It was quite plain that she was telling me it would be less trouble if I let Trish die. And that was true. If Trish died, we would all have an easier life, but that's not what Trish wanted, and I was speaking for her. Incidentally, Trish and the duty nurse were listening to this conversation. The doctor's comment upset me, and I felt her loyalty had been given to the management of the home and not to her patient. I was still

---

21 A decade later when the government had hinted during the pandemic that the elderly should be excluded from treatment, I too found myself being "let go". Before that I had been under the impression that the duty of care had improved. NHS changes had been dramatic from 2010 to 2020.

thinking about things when she followed up with a remark that did not make sense: "If you do anything that affects the neck you could hurt her, and I would have to refer the matter to an assessment team of up to eight people."

Now this was like a red rag to the bull. Here she was, in effect, telling me to let Trish die but if I tried anything to save her, it would be a disaster. *What, I thought, was worse than dying?* She then listed all the experts who would be set on to me if I did anything. They included social workers, neurologists, Parkinson's specialists, physios, nutritionists et alia.

I then chirped up rather stupidly. "You have forgotten the most important expert of the lot."

"No, I don't think I have forgotten anyone".

"Yes, you have," I retorted. "How about a professor of Logic or Humanity?"

That made her very angry.

"Don't you be condescending to me! Apart from anything else, you are going to upset my career."

Now that was the wrong thing to say to me. I just turned my back on her and walked away. The nurse who had witnessed the incident was trapped behind her desk; she was trying to look as small as possible.

What the doctor and I did not know at that stage was that there was an answer to dropped-head syndrome. As a layperson, I could not have been expected to know about it, but perhaps she should have been more considerate towards me and investigated the condition in her own medical world. Eventually, I stumbled on an answer by experiment. When I had tackled the problem, a team was sent to keep me in my place.

It is at this stage in my writing that I should say something about the medical relationships between the qualified nurse in the nursing home, the local doctor's surgery and the hospital. For as I write this, we are in the middle of the second Covid lockdown. The death rate in care homes has been high from Covid, but I would ask the question: "How many deaths were caused by bad social care and NHS organisations, compounded and hidden under the Covid blanket?"[22]

There was one qualified nurse supported by a variable number of care assistants in the home. A few of the carers were well experienced, but many were very young, and some had difficulty with the English language. The young sat at a computer and ticked boxes. When the forms were completed, the nursing assistants were qualified. As I found on occasions, an eighteen-year-old could then be in charge of critically ill patients overnight. A significant number of the carers were themselves stressed but hid their problems because they needed the money. Some went home to

---

22 The concern was eventually examined in the Covid inquiry in 2023.

care for elderly relatives.

The nurse was well qualified but many of her qualifications could not be used in a care home. A local doctor came in once a week to guide the nurse and write prescriptions. But the doctor was busy with her own surgery and was very reluctant to attend the home outside her routine visits. Thus, many minor problems were solved by calling for an ambulance, taking the patient to hospital, and returning him or her by ambulance later in the day. That was to become a big issue in 2020 and, in my view, spread Covid throughout the care homes. The process put a strain on everyone. These standard procedures were obviously not good when we were going into a pandemic, and maybe this was one of the reasons for the high death rate in care homes.

It is well known that Parkinson sufferers can have significant problems going to the toilet. So it was with Trish. There was an occasion when she had not gone to the toilet for the best part of a week. I examined her stomach to find hard lumps pushing up under the skin and asked if she could be given an enema. She had diverticulitis and was in pain. Everyone was busy—as usual—and I was told the nurse could not do that without a visit and a prescription from the doctor. However, the doctor would not be visiting for some days and then the prescription had to be fetched. It could be that Trish might not be helped to go to the toilet for some ten days overall. That was totally unacceptable, and I said so.

I told Trish that there was a problem. I asked her, "Trish, can I get close and personal to see if I can solve things?"

She was desperate and would have agreed to anything at this stage. So, on went the rubber gloves and some gel. The first "cannonball" was the most difficult but, after it was removed, the next was easy and then there was an eruption. I looked at Trish and felt pleased but embarrassed. My embarrassment faded when she said, "Oh, thank you, thank you! The pain has gone."

I told the nurse Trish had been to the toilet. She looked at me strangely. The incident was repeated some weeks later and the message got out. But from then on, a prescription was kept in the home. I had beaten the system.

However, my previous clash with the doctor led to an unexpected development.

Chapter Seventeen
I Treat Dropped-Head Syndrome

My answer to the head drop was simple and logical. I reckoned if we couldn't find a therapeutic solution with a collar, then the answer was to lift the whole head to release the jaw sufficiently to chew. We were doing this manually. I would stand behind Trish with my hands round her forehead while a carer fed her or vice versa. So why not make a device to do the same in a bed or chair? The first experiment was a baseball cap reversed, with pulleys on the back of the hat and bed, and a jammer as used on dinghies to hold any adjustment. It worked but it was uncomfortable, even with some sponge at the front of the hat. While my experiment was taking place, the home was vehement that they would have nothing to do with me, and the nurse and carers were told to keep clear of the room.

At mealtimes, food for Trish was left out in the corridor and I was left to do all the feeding. It was now that I brought more cooking utensils into the room for mixing and preparing food. The management went ballistic, and I was ordered to remove everything, but

I refused. The company's headquarters put their lawyers on me, but I still said no. They said they would take me to court, and I said I would be delighted to meet them there. That didn't happen because I knew too much, and they didn't want the publicity.

Eventually, I set up the lifting device with a woman's firmly-fitting felt hat and got the thumbs-up from Trish. Over the weeks that followed, Trish ate and her weight was maintained and even started to improve. Then two fantastic things happened. Firstly, she started to talk to me again. I had learnt with Trish that the hat was good for about forty-five minutes, then slowly I could reduce some of the pressure and keep it on while she slept. If I did this, of course, I never left her side. The final improvement was that as I removed the hat each time, her jaw stayed away from her chest and the ulceration, which I was now tending to myself, healed and disappeared. She could also now watch TV again and I would sit with her in the bed; we would talk and watch TV together. The device was refined and could be moved from bed to chair and wheelchair. Far from just being a feeding device, it was also therapeutic. I made a video about its use and wrote a paper, which were used to convince interested experts.

But still the home would have nothing to do with me. That is, until a physiotherapist came to teach me how to stretch and massage aching limbs. She saw what I was doing and supported me. She also told me there had been similar progress in America, and she knew a charity that would help me. The charity was called REMAP and their aim was to support the NHS with unusual devices for the disabled.

The assessment team that had been actioned by the care home's doctor came and met me on site. They had read my paper and the Parkinson's nurse had already discussed my progress with the neurologist, who had given his approval. Far from damaging the nerves in the neck, the slow change during feeding was good for the nerves. At the beginning of the meeting, I took them to see Trish, who was sitting up. Her eyes were wide open and she said good afternoon to the team. That was a real shock for them.

We left Trish and went back to the meeting room where one of the members stood up and said, "Ladies and gentlemen, sometimes we can get so focused on our routines that it takes someone like Mr Adcock to shake us by thinking laterally."

I received a pat on the back and they departed. I did not see the doctor again, but I understand she had time off to have a baby. That was a good arrangement.

The head-lifter was now accepted by the system as a good idea, and Trish's head even stayed away from her chest. However, the home still did not accept the situation until a doctor from REMAP came to visit me. He asked me to join the charity and said he would insure me for my work. I thought, *What work?*

It soon became clear that there were many people in the locality that had a similar problem to Trish's, and I was wanted to travel with a physiotherapist and make devices for others. What a turnaround!

The first client had heard I was coming, and I am sure she expected a magician. Her condition was not as bad as Trish's and her main concern was that she wanted to watch television. I made a couple of visits and TV was watched again, but I realised I could not cope with the expectations. I told the REMAP doctor I would help from a distance. After all, the device had been accepted and there needed to be a more professional approach; my device needed to be manufactured properly and developed for people living with the syndrome.

Once things were accepted and I was insured, the care home reluctantly agreed I could train the staff so they could use the head-lifter to feed Trish. However, problems just mounted up. The home became very short-staffed and a small kitchen that was used to prepare foods for nursed patients was closed down. I could not get the right food preparation for Trish, so I brought in mixers and a microwave oven. The manager was far from happy, but my view was that if *they* could not cope then *I* would and, as far as I was concerned, the duty of care had been passed to me.

Chapter Eighteen
I Decide to Sell the Family House

When the estate agent visited me in Dales Drive in September and said, "I can sell your house," it seemed a good idea. It was certainly in my mind that Trish would never be coming home to the bungalow with its big garden, and it was not the right place for me to live on my own.

I replied, "Do it by Christmas and you have a deal."

Looking at the longer term, it was certainly a good thing to do. But what I had not thought through were the short-term implications and, above all, I did not consider the unexpected actions of the people I was dealing with. I did not know it then, but I was about to find out who was going to make life very difficult and who was going to help and sympathise with me when, like Alice, the hole I found myself falling into just got bigger and bigger.

I had, however, considered the problems surrounding Trish and knew winter was going to be a struggle for her. I remembered back to Christmas 2011 and the fight I had had to keep her air passage open through a period of infection. In the back of my mind, any move had to be to a ground-floor flat, because my relationship with the care home had broken down and I wanted the option to take Trish out of the care home for the last weeks of her life. A move, therefore, had to be swift and it had to be over before the darkest days of winter.

The house move started really well. Within twelve hours of the bungalow going on the market I had accepted an offer and, in the following twenty-four hours, I had found a flat I liked. I made an offer, and it was accepted. The move would be as fast as the solicitor could spell "conveyance". I had confidence because my buyer had all but completed the deal on his own sale, and his new job and the children's school were within walking distance of the bungalow. They were naturally keen to have Christmas in their new home and have the children settled before the beginning of the new term. My vendors had also found a house they wanted, and they told me that, if there were problems, they would find temporary accommodation with their parents. I felt there was substance to my expectations.

It was very good news that the move would go so quickly because the dark cloud over the care home grew blacker and very difficult problems were building up. I had been coping with care home problems for nearly three years and it just meant I would have to be more dedicated and tenacious in caring for and protecting Trish. So, my work rate would increase. I would just have to cope while I was down-sizing and cleaning.

My personal activities went out of the window, and I started to lose some contact with family and friends. Perhaps my optimism was somewhat premature.

When the solicitor started to make nervous statements about Christmas and the vendor asked for a little time (talk of moving to parents was now forgotten!), I knew I was falling faster into the hole. Nevertheless, I decided to continue with the sale. I had given my word to my buyer and money in the bank would give me the ammunition to continue moving. I sold the bungalow in early December and moved into my small motorhome and camped on a local touring-site to wait for the flat to become vacant.

Almost as soon as I had made the decision to move to the touring-site, the nursing in the care home became a shambles. Relationships between caring staff and management hit an all-time low and staff started leaving. There were many times when there were only one or two carers to look after twenty people. The pressure on the remaining carers caused even the youngsters to leave. Frequently there would be only one nurse on duty to cover all the residents (more than fifty in number), including those being nursed. I really had to care for Trish almost full time, because

I knew otherwise she would be left for hours on her own.

Once in the motorhome I was warm and comfortable, but I was awake at 6 a.m. and went out into the cold to shower. In the first few weeks it rained and rained and rained. Luckily, the site was quite well drained, but managing the motorhome was a task on its own in the adverse conditions. It was heaven to break my journey to Trish and get into the warmth of Costa to have coffee and toast and to talk to new friends. After coffee the problems started.

I arrived at the care home at about 8 a.m. to see Trish. She would invariably be waiting, unable to move, with her eyes partially open and filled with fluid. The routine was always the same. A hug, then, "Morning, Trish. Cup of tea?"

When she could, I would get a positive response. On good days it would be

"Oh, yes please" or a squeeze of the hand. But things went from bad to worse and the CQC became involved.

Unfortunately, the good days were over. I sat her up, cleaned her eyes and she just looked at me as though she was glad to see someone. I made her tea, but she did not drink very much, and I realised she was getting a cold. My heart sank as I remembered the previous Christmas. It was a year on, and she was yet weaker. Were those eyes still telling me to fight on, or were they telling me it was over?

Everything was getting so very desperate. I closed my mind to the dilemma and knew I must try to feed her.

Until this stage, some of the experienced carers and I had managed to maintain Trish's weight at around five stone, but now I knew that—if the cold got a hold—Trish would not be able to eat much. In any case, the home had also lost its capability to prepare food and feed someone like Trish. The remaining few, now relatively inexperienced, carers did not have time to feed people over an extended mealtime. Trish and those like her were becoming an encumbrance to the management of a private company. In financial terms, it was best that patients depart the home one way or another while management hid issues and reorganised. I had already watched people die early, and unnecessarily, of malnutrition (in my judgement) and no one had the right to do that to Trish. The fight would continue on my terms, even if the result was going to be the same.

Tina, also, now understood some of the shortcomings of the home and wrote to the manager about nutrition. As an expert in nutrition and caring for the disabled, Tina had some effect, but the home wouldn't, or couldn't, correct the major problems to do with manning, training, nursing of the elderly, and respecting the patients' dignity.

The nursing department was some way away from the main part of the home and, in the past, in order to cope with food and its preparation, there was a small kitchen close by with a fridge, microwave oven, dishwasher and drinking-water from the tap. This made sense, but with a shortage of staff it became unhygienic and was closed. This meant everything came from the main kitchen, where the chef literally drew a line on the floor to confine carers to a tiny area where they queued to prepare food for those being nursed. I was immediately barred from the main kitchen and was told to ask a carer to fetch food. As the main kitchen was 100 yards away, the round trip to get a glass of water was 200 yards. Of course, with insufficient staff to manage a small kitchen, the change was chaotic. I was fighting for every calorie put into Trish's mouth, but I was not going to be thwarted. So, I bought a fridge, microwave oven, food processor, sieve and kettle. I bought food from Waitrose and prepared highly puréed food myself. In any case, this was only a step on from what I had been doing when there was a functioning kitchen.

Predictably, the manager told me to move everything out. I was quoted fire, mayhem, health and safety, and duty of care. If there was anything guaranteed to wind me up, it was for them to start chanting these over-used mantras. I just said, "No."

The manager then quoted company headquarters' policy and I said, "No."

The manager suggested that I might like to move my wife to another home, and she reported me to the primary care trust (PCT).

Trish's breathing was now awful, and I was clearing her nose and throat at regular intervals, something the nurses and carers would not do because it was considered to be invasive![23] Because I was worried about Trish's breathing, I was now coming back into the home late into the night and, when I found my way back through the rain to the motorhome, I fell onto my bed quite exhausted.

Now, if I thought my hole was black and deep and could not get worse, it did in fact get worse; in amongst my caring tasks, I was forever on the phone to get a proper roof over my head. Slowly, the truth was dawning that my vendor was having difficulty and was uncomfortable at the thought of any disturbance over Christmas and the New Year. Back came the message that they would even like to delay until March! The solicitor was also beginning to suck her teeth and she told me about the conveyance on a flat being difficult. She was due to leave work the day before Christmas Eve and not return until the New Year. The PCT was

---

23 Caring rules in a care home were made very restrictive by the NHS. You could smell the fear of litigation. But the rules were not always helpful to the patients.

sympathetic about my problems with the care home but they suggested that, for Trish's sake, I should consider moving her. The last "good news" was that the touring-site was closing for a month for maintenance and the only other site was flooded.

Of course, much of my hole was of my own making, but people were now throwing dirt in from the top. Was I ever going to get out?

At about this point—when I knew I was homeless and my wife was dying—I could have been forgiven for having a nervous breakdown and giving in, but instead I went on the attack. I reported the care home to the Care Quality Commission (CQC)—something I should have done before—and wrote articles, which went to fellow sympathisers and the PCT. I visited every estate agent in Wimborne and re-evaluated my decision on the flat. The cavalry, in the form of my family, also arrived and together we reviewed the care home situation. There was also probably some concern about my sanity.

Christmas came and it was almost a non-event for me. I watched TV and saw people in silly hats giving instruction about food and presents, and felt I was looking at the TV from another planet a million miles away. However, it wasn't all bad, because I visited Tina for Christmas Eve supper and declared that, come what may, I would find a way to take Trish to Christmas lunch with John, Kate and family.

Chapter Nineteen
Christmas 2012

The act of moving Trish was not easy on Christmas Day, but I knew she was keen because, when I asked her if she would like to visit some of her family, her eyes opened wide, and I got a very distinct nod of approval. Despite everything that was happening to her, she seemed to want to live and enjoy her family.

The care home was not too happy about my plan to take Trish out for the day, and they left me to wash and dress her, and get together the paraphernalia to prepare her food. It was not too difficult getting her into the car for she was now so light, but I had to be very gentle and careful not to hurt her. I packed duvets and pillows round her to keep her warm. I was glad to see John waiting at the house and we did not bother with the wheelchair. John carried his mum all the way like a baby in his arms and laid her in a chair in the lounge. Trish normally slept most of the time, but her eyes stayed open and followed the family all day. I reduced the Christmas meal virtually to liquid, and she ate slowly. Amazingly, she was still awake when I took her back to the home, but by the time she was ready for bed I knew she would sleep deeply that night. I lay down and cuddled her and she did indeed go into a deep sleep. The day out had been worthwhile.

Looking back, it was the last significant event in her life. I am glad we, her family, had made the effort.

As I went to sleep that night, I reflected on all those people who were in a similar situation in care homes and had to lie, very lonely, just staring at the ceiling. I also had recurring thoughts about frightened children trying to get warm and sleep in Syria, which at that time was in a mess. My family was so lucky! I resolved to get up in the morning and sort things out. It was certainly not a time to whinge and moan.

Unfortunately, I could do very little. The UK was shut for Christmas and the New Year. We had established that there were no vacancies elsewhere for Trish. The only remaining options were to leave Trish where she was and protect her, or move her to a new abode with me. The latter option was also fading, unless it was into the motorhome. However, the estate agents were open for business between the two holidays, so I could review my offer on the flat.

Eventually, I found a couple of options that would do as accommodation. I made provisional offers, and they were accepted. I was totally honest and kept them all informed of my primary choice. I then went back to my vendor and told him that the delay was causing heartache and financial problems. He was keen not to lose the sale, so I explained that my touring-site was closing and the alternative was flooded. I was going to have to move into a hotel and my costs would increase. I now needed something much more positive, or I was off. He agreed to pay my hotel bill, but that was soon changed to half the bill and, when it was paid, he *only* made a £200 contribution. He said Christmas was costly and difficult. How I would have liked to change my difficulties for his!

The rain stopped.

While I was in the hotel, I looked at the alternative campsite. It was drying out, but the bad news was the weather was forecast to become exceptionally cold and snow was coming. Strangely, the site was quite busy, but the ladies who ran it made room for me. At last, I had somewhere to go after the week in the hotel.

Trish was now very poorly and eating very little. Although I was spending long hours with her, I was no longer achieving very much, apart from making sure she was warm and comfortable and cuddling her when I saw that silent tear fall down her cheek. That really hurt.

Chapter Twenty
Professional Support Is Awful

Well, the temperature dropped, and the snow fell. Trish now had chest and urinary infections that caused a fever, and she stopped eating. Things were now serious; the hole I had fallen into now seemed to be an abyss. Trish was going to die, and I was camping. The snow fell and added to my problems, and I was beginning to feel ill with the same chest infection that was affecting Trish. It was at this stage I hit a personal low. My own health was under serious threat and was going to be a problem in the months and years that followed.

It had snowed heavily and, in the morning, I had to get help to get my car off the campsite. Once out on the back road I rolled down a hill, only to be confronted by a tree that had fallen across the road. I got out of the car to look at the problem and realised I was stuck. I knew I could not get back up the hill in the snow. That was for sure. As I stood there wondering what to do, a very loud crack sounded. Strangely, there was such an echo over the dull snow that, for a moment, I didn't know which tree it was. Luckily, it was a tree behind the hedge that had fallen on the snow with a crash.

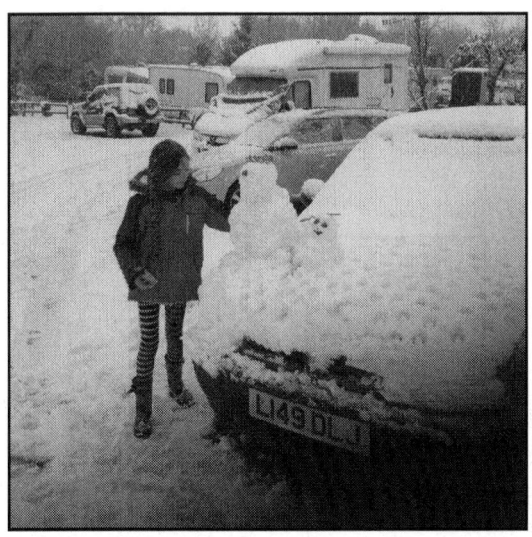

Girl playing. My motorhome is in the background.

Never mind, I thought, *I'll get my smartphone out of my pocket and get help from the campsite.* It was at this stage I really felt the world was against me because my phone was locked and unusable. The tree in front of me was big and rested on boughs with leaves filling the gaps. I was now angry. I had to get to Trish.

I backed the car as best I could on the ice and drove at the tree. I was angry. Very, very angry! As luck would have it, I burst through between the branches without hitting the trunk. I reached the care home and rang the campsite. By nightfall the tree had been sawn up and removed.

Again, I went on the attack. It was mid-January. I told the seller he had until midday the following day to exchange contracts and I wanted completion within the following four days. In fairness, my vendor now had a genuine problem that was affecting the exchange. His solicitor was a sole practitioner and was seriously ill, but frankly I no longer cared about other people's problems. It was midday or nothing. A peripatetic solicitor was found and struggled to travel in the snow, but I did not care. My own solicitor "broke the rules" and shouldered the financial risk of the debilitated solicitor. Eight minutes before my deadline, contracts were exchanged and we headed to completion as I had demanded. Trish had eaten nothing for over two weeks and as we approached 25th January, when I took charge of the keys to the flat, Trish had not had anything to drink for a week and it was not for lack of effort on my part.

As I cared for Trish over the twelve years she had Parkinson's, I had learnt not to be surprised at stupid policies and crazy organisation in the NHS and the care home, but while Trish was becoming ill with infections it became quite obvious she needed antibiotics. The medicine was delivered but Trish could not swallow. I tried to give her the medicines but I was failing, so I turned to the nurse and said, "Could you please arrange for Trish to have the antibiotics injected or fed to her via a drip?"

She simply replied, "It is not policy to do that in a care home."

I insisted that the duty doctor attend, and I asked *him* to do it but he refused. He also kept talking about Trish's "terminal condition" while she was listening, and I could see from Trish's face that this was the last nail in her coffin. I tried to wave down his crass insensitivity, but he didn't understand. He said he could move her to hospital, but to transfer her in the cold and, after his indiscretion, would just kill her cruelly. What was this duty of care that was so easily mouthed? I refused his offer and said I would take full charge of any drugs and drip-feed them into Trish's throat with a one-millilitre syringe. They then had the audacity to make *me* sign a risk assessment form.

Why did I do what I did? Well, in my opinion, it was not for the system to turn off my wife's life; that was down to my understanding of her wishes. I had known her for sixty years and I had her Enduring Power of Attorney. Perhaps I was being unreasonable, but I could not just walk away; I still wanted to fight for Trish.

I was now coughing for long periods and had pains in my chest, and I felt sorry for both of us.

When Friday 25th January arrived, I collected the keys to the flat, but could not get my goods and chattels out of storage until the following Monday. I was enveloped in a nightmare!

The family became concerned for both of us. Lesley came up from Devon. I left the campsite and camped in the flat. There was nothing I could do for Trish. Lesley and I took it in turns to comfort her. I went to see my doctor who reassured me about Trish, and now it was my turn for antibiotics.

On Monday 28th, the furniture arrived, with my family. I did my best to help with the unpacking, but when my bed was made I was glad to see the old friend and just fell into it. I slept for some hours then got up to see Trish. I was aware the end was in sight. At midnight I climbed into bed with her and held her head in the crook of my elbow. I did not feel well but she relaxed totally, and we slept.

At three o'clock I awoke with some discomfort in my chest. I felt all the little bones in Trish's neck ripple and crack; then I felt her neck go soft and her jaw drop. As far as I was concerned, Mr Parkinson had just departed and had ceased to hold her muscles rigid. I was glad to see the back of him.

Perhaps I shouldn't write this, but I was glad it was over. If I had died at the same time, I would have been happy. However, I went back to my flat and the bed.

Within the hour, the phone rang and Lesley told me that her mum had been formally pronounced dead, but I knew she had died in my arms.

During this period and all the difficult time afterwards, my family was marvellous to me. Now I had to remember they were suffering in their own ways with their own loss. In contemplating this event, more than ever I believe that no one should have to die alone. My experience in the care home was that I had just gone through a relatively rare event. I had made friends with so many elderly people during my time in the home and I had watched them deteriorate and die alone.

During this awful period of moving into the flat, Tina went round the other neighbouring flats and explained my situation. I received sympathy and support from all my new neighbours, except one. Rather than talking to me, that one person complained to property management who, in turn, wrote to me to tell me to move my motorhome off the site. At the time there was lots of parking space, so I assumed the occupant of this one flat just didn't like the look of my small motorhome. All I wanted to do was grieve and unpack. I spoke to the property management and gave them my thoughts, but there was no reply. I eventually left a note for the complaining flat-owner to ask her to talk to me, but she and the property management just walked round me and left me to my own devices ... probably a good thing.

Chapter Twenty-One
Trish Dies

During the last few weeks of Trish's life my family had talked to the care home management and had been offended by their condescension and lack of understanding. In turn, they told me they understood why my relationship with the care home was strained.

After Trish died early that morning, my family emptied everything out of her room within an hour because they knew I would never want to go back. I did, however, go back at the weekend when I knew I would only see carers and nurses, and I was able to say thank you to those who actually cared.

The CQC *did* carry out an assessment and the PCT passed my notes up through their line management. The home had to make changes to their manning and shift system. I understand that, also, limitations were put on their contracts with the NHS and Social Services, for I was not alone with critical comments. Finally, the nursing department was closed down. Supposedly it was for building renovation but that—for me—was just a cover story. However, it did re-open later.

Trish would have been pleased to know just how

many people came to the funeral. The seats were full and people were standing in the aisles. I stood up at the end of the service, thanked everyone, and said how I thought that throughout such a long period of caring, Trish and I had become invisible but I had been wrong. A lot of people had remembered.

OK, my bad thoughts at a difficult time were over. I walked home from Costa after my long period of reminiscing that morning. I had lain in bed watching the shaft of early morning light. I continued to go to Costa and "my other family" consoled me.

Chapter Twenty-Two
The Lady Upstairs

When Trish died and I had rid myself of the chest infection, I thought I was going to close the flat door and let the rest of my life drift by. There was little I could see positive about the future. Checks for cancer had done nothing other than to bring me an infection.

Towards the end of the first year after Trish died, I was feeling somewhat lonely and depressed. In addition, I was being given a really hard time by the occupant of an upstairs flat who had never forgiven me for unloading my luggage in the parking area close to the flats during the awful winter the year before.

There was, however, some good news because a lady in the flat above me was watching and, unbeknown to me, was sympathetic about what had happened over the previous months.

My flat, having its own door and garage, is somewhat remote from the main building and the other seven flats, but I have to go into the main hall to collect the post. That is where I first met Mary Brightwell. We introduced ourselves and started chatting; the chat soon became uninhibited for an early meeting.

Eventually, Mary said she had Parkinson's. Of course, my experience of caring for Trish was discussed and eventually I said, "I hope you don't mind me asking… do you have a close friend or member of the family to help you through the bad times?"

Mary replied, "My son lives in London, and he visits me once a month."

I replied quite cheekily, "I was thinking more of a day-to-day relationship. As Parkinson's progresses, what you don't want is a lonely struggle."

I was not intending to volunteer, but it might have sounded that way. I was just genuinely concerned about future developments for someone with a disease I had learned so much about.

We passed from time to time and spoke generally about things. I slowly became aware of her interest in nature and that she wanted some assistance to do some gardening in the communal garden. I volunteered and helped with tools and the odd heavy task. The upshot of this was that we would talk, and sometimes I would make her a cup of tea, which was easy for me with my downstairs flat virtually on the edge of the garden. As we talked, the one thing that was apparent was that we had both travelled the world, but that was almost the end of our similar past activities. However, we were both intrigued by the dissimilarities in our pasts.

Mary had been an English teacher and lecturer with a great interest in the arts, music and theatre. She was also a pacifist. She was everything I was not. We were able to swap experiences and points of view that would have been so difficult in years past. We did not stop talking and drinking tea, or even the odd glass of wine. Now with such interest in one another and Mary living in a flat close by, our relationship was likely to progress but there was a misconception on both sides; for Mary saw me going out with Geraldine, an old friend of Trish's, to play golf and Mary would enter the garden with Brian, from Devon, who would supply her with plants when he visited at the weekend. Both of us saw our relationship as tea and sympathy and no more. Then things changed.

Despite our initial misreading of one another's situation, we were actually, and unbelievably at our time of life, falling in love. Slowly we learnt from one another that our friendships with Geraldine and Brian were just that; they were friendships and there was no other arrangement. Then there were two events that caused a big change.

When Tom came from London, he and his mother had been in the habit of playing golf, but Mary was finding that—as the months went by—Parkinson's was putting an end to that. So, she asked me if I would take him to my club on his next visit. This I did. I also organised a buggy, so Mary could come with us. We all got on well and Tom hinted that he would like to do it again. Still, little was said about our relationship. However, I learned later that Mary was looking out for me as I travelled to and from the flat—and when she was in the garden I was there too. Our mutual attraction was becoming obvious to us both.

Soon afterwards, we were both invited to a party at Mary's friend's house. It was a cold, dark winter's night, and I said I would walk her to the party. I drank some wine and chatted to various neighbours, then I noticed Mary sitting quietly on the settee. I realised she was looking at me in that special way that is so meaningful. Our eyes met and we both understood.

After an appropriate length of time, Mary stood up and excused herself. People around understood that her Parkinson's created limitations and I quite naturally said I would walk her back to her flat. There were no objections to our early departure; everyone seemed to understand. Once outside the door I turned to Mary and said something along the lines of, "I think it is time that we just got on with things."

There was no answer, just pressure, as she hooked her arm into mine and we strode purposefully into the dark. I could feel her smiling.

The easiest route to her flat was through my backdoor and I asked her if she would like a cup of tea. She accepted. (I have subsequently learned Mary is not that keen on tea, but at this early stage she never refused.)

Mary was just standing watching me put water in the kettle and get out some cups when she whispered something I could not hear. Bugger my hearing! I said sorry and asked Mary to repeat herself.

Mary said, "I need a hug."

My mind was on tea-making, but I duly complied. We drank tea and Mary never made it to her flat.

The years have passed, and we have never spent a night apart—except when I spent nights in hospital or she visited her family. More about that later.

After that eventful night, we started a new life and began to make plans. We began with a week in one flat then a week in the other, which caused much confusion as we never knew where things were.

"The milk is in the fridge upstairs."

"Have you seen my glasses?" and so on.

We just had to decide. Mary's flat had some advantages, but it was upstairs. My flat was downstairs, had more storage space, its own door and a garage. So, *my flat* was the preferred option. There was a big cost-saving on living together and we could get rid of a car. In any case, Mary was already not very committed to driving. Then came the big question and Mary was first to mutter it over supper.

"Shall we get married?"

It was getting close to a proposal although the ball had just been hit into my court.

"Oops, Mary! Go no further. I'm a bit old-fashioned. If there is a question to ask, I will ask it."

I left the subject hanging over us for a few days, but I *did* ask, and we became engaged. We both knew where we were going and, by then, it was no longer a surprise. However, it *was* a surprise for our families and their reactions surprised us. However, we should have expected the unexpected.

Mary's son, Tom, seemed to be protective but not entirely displeased. He had obviously taken a view about some of Mary's past boyfriends and was keen that she should get it right this time. He wanted a very positive period of engagement and I had to explain to him that it was not like young love with a lifetime to plan and get things right. In any case, it was impossible to see into the future. We were on a cliff edge and had to get on with things before we fell off. He then interviewed me and asked me about an exit strategy. I explained there was only one exit, and we would make wills. I could see he was uneasy, but he understood. Once decisions were made, he appeared supportive.

When my family was told, they too were supportive. Well, the eldest three certainly were but my younger son had reservations that I did not know about or understand. Things came to a head when Mary decided to sell her flat. We had talked about various options but, in the end, it was obviously down to Mary. The flat was sold, and Mary decided to keep some of the cash to provide for any care she might need as Parkinson's advanced. The rest she gave to Tom towards his eventual family home.

It was then that Mark wrote long e-mails calling "foul" and that is what I did not understand. What Mary did with her property had nothing to do with my family or me, especially as Mary's property had been financed largely by her ex-husband on the understanding that his son would be the eventual beneficiary. I tried to see my son to discuss the problem, but he was always "busy" and eventually I had to accept his message, which was loud and clear. He had largely abandoned his mother and now, for sure, I was abandoned too. As the years have gone by, I have grieved over the loss of contact with my son and his family. After communicating on WhatsApp, I still did not understand.

Chapter Twenty-Three
Married Again: a Five-Year Contract

We were married in Wimborne Town Hall on 5 April 2014 and had a family gathering at a restaurant a few doors away. The whole event went well, supported in one way or another by other family members. In fairness, Mark in his professional role managed other family members to take photos that Tina and Mo constructed into a lovely album.

So, we were married and went to Verona and Venice for our honeymoon. This enabled us to visit John and family while Izzy (my youngest granddaughter) took part in an international windsurfing competition on Lake Garda. It was the start of her progression to becoming National Champion and rising high up in international competition.

In April 2014 Mary and I were established as man and wife; we were both deliriously happy with the decisions we had made, but knew there would be some problems. I was ten years older than Mary and had been continually chased for possible cardiovascular and prostate problems, which I had not taken very seriously. It had been fourteen years since Mary was diagnosed with Parkinson's. We joked that our marriage could be no more than a five-year contract, but it was no joke, more an acceptance of reality. I know people thought, *Why is he doing this when he has gone through it all before? After all, he lost his first wife to the ravages of Parkinson's.* Well, I knew what I was doing and, when you love someone, you cope with the downside. In any case, things were to develop differently from expectations: I was going to need Mary at least as much as she was going to need me.

When we married, Mary said, "We have so much history but none together."

After a few years, history built up very quickly. We had great holidays in Madeira and Quiberon, but then decided that travelling abroad was full of hassle and we should stay in the UK. Consequently, we had a wonderful cruise around the Scottish islands.

A new pattern of travel emerged after we purchased a new car. The back seats came out of the new brown Yeti, and it was adapted for picnicking and B&B travel. Then came a small caravan and, later, a more powerful Yeti and a bigger caravan.

At home we fell into a routine. I adapted to Mary's friends with time away in Devon. Mary met my friends too, and so we formed our own history.

All went well to begin with, but then my own health conditions created clouds on the horizon.

From the start, my deafness was an issue. This was more than annoying. Mary quite often had to say things several times before we understood one another. If I had been on the receiving end of such irritation, I think I would have gone up the wall, but Mary's patience was—and still is—amazing. Then came shingles, which caused pain and irritation for a year or so and caused me to walk the floor through the night. Then followed the passing of very fine kidney stones, which was very painful for a few days but the problem went away. Then a hernia, which I live with still. Later, after a third biopsy, I was diagnosed with prostate cancer. I decided to live with that too and not have treatment. I am still living with it and know that one day it may get the better of me. Things became complicated during the pandemic when treatment became difficult.

Chapter Twenty-Four
My Cardiac Sky

Since I was seventeen, I have been chased by the medics for high blood pressure and a heart murmur. The murmur was eventually dismissed as technology advanced, but like most people of my age I was on statins, and they were to cause all sorts of problems.

It was ironic that Rowlands Hill, Wimborne, which my doctor had used in an example of a patient whom he had buried, became my nemesis. His threat of a stroke arising out of a stressful life had caused me to retire from work some nineteen years before; caring for Trish had added to stress levels. What followed was almost inevitable.

One very cold February morning as I was walking up Rowlands Hill—with traffic at a standstill and pumping out noxious fumes—I started to feel aches in my back and arms. I knew what was happening but thought it would go away. The aches eased when I entered our flat, but Mary sensed I was distressed. I told her I had some small aches and pains but would not go to the doctor because it was trivial. Mary broke down in tears and thrust the phone into my hand. What I didn't realise at the time was that those tears probably saved my life. I explained to the receptionist at my GP's surgery why I needed an appointment and was given one straightaway. History was building fast and we were only halfway through our "contract".

The nurse tut-tutted as the paper came out of the ECG. "I will need to talk to the doctor about this."

That started a train of events over the next two years. First came the diagnosis from an angiogram with a wire in my leg to my heart: I had advanced cardiovascular disease. I was offered open-heart surgery, but I suggested stents would suit me better for, impatient as ever, I could not afford a long recovery. The first two stents went, as part of research, into the right side of my heart. After I recovered, two more would go into the left. I won't say that the first session was painful; it was interesting. I spent my time talking to the surgeon, doctor and nurse about their tasks, and watched the results on an overhead screen. It was great teamwork and was all very straight forward.

Two months went by. I felt a little better but could not walk well uphill. So, I returned for the final two stents. Now I was an old hand. It was the third time the wire had entered my body and wriggled its way up to my heart. I again chatted away to the team. I was even flirting with the nurse and lady doctor.

Then the strangest event took place. I was chatting away, and it was as though someone had just changed the TV channel. There I was, looking at a really blue sky and little puffy white clouds. I was flying, eighteen again, in my Harvard, and rolling it round the clouds. It was so very peaceful and so very enjoyable.

In fact, I was dying.

Then my peace was shattered, and I was extremely annoyed at the disturbance. There was a banging noise, and I felt a painful rigidity in my whole body. (That was the electric shock.) Then followed a chaotic noise and I was back on the planet. People were talking very loudly around me. Somebody slapped my face. Something was put over my nose and mouth. I remembered that feeling, but I was not in my jet! It was a medical mask.

"Are you all right, Mr Adcock? We have had a minor problem."

"I'm fine."

I lied because I was very annoyed to leave my peaceful sky. They also lied. It was not a minor problem. I had been to the edge of the cliff and back again.

After the fourth stent had been put in place, an artery had split. Blood had stopped going to my brain and the heart sac started to fill with blood. The team now went into top gear to fit a fifth stent that would stop the bleeding before my chest filled with blood. They must have accomplished the task very quickly, but I was not going home as soon as planned. I was well wired up in a ward for the night.

Although Mary had her own problems, she had to help me recover, which I did, slowly but surely. I now walk up and down Rowlands Hill daily, in the knowledge I have the better of it but also knowing that it will still be there long after I have gone. Now when I look at a blue sky and summer clouds I say with some pride, "That's my cardiac sky."

I have always known death is inevitable. I have now experienced the peace that can come with it. In the meantime, I am following Churchill's philosophy of KBO (keep buggering on). Luck is still my shadow!

Chapter Twenty-Five
Old Age and Health Issues

After another marriage and surviving a cardiac arrest, it would have been reasonable to finish my writing with a happy ending, but life was to continue, and the world would continue to go round while spitting out problems for humanity, and humanity also causing problems for humanity. Mary and I were going to enjoy our life together while fighting the problems of old age. It was, and still is, a fight, but we fulfilled our five-year contract with ease.

At this stage in my writing, Mary has had Parkinson's for some twenty-one years. The pattern of her illness is much the same as it was; her past life and fitness have been of benefit. The drugs have had to be adjusted from time to time, but Mary has continued to think she can do anything. Unfortunately, the reduction in dopamine saps her strength and takes that thought away. During those periods I have to help her. What has been amazing is that I have successfully encouraged her to eat. However, Mary is prone to falling. Bad falls have landed her in hospital but, with training, her walking has improved.

Unfortunately, the danger of serious falls will always be a problem.

We used to love walking along Poole Beach. During a walk one brilliantly sunny day, the wind blew, and her endless trails of tissue paper became a problem. She dropped a tissue and chased it. She recovered the flying devil but turned and fell. Her arm went down, which dislocated her shoulder, and her head hit the ground. Dyskinesia set in and she shook her dislocated limb causing much pain. I lay on the ground with her to stop her gyrations. A crowd gathered and the dogs came to smell us. I could not use my phone, but a spectator kindly rang 999.

In the hospital I helped to put her shoulder back in place and her head was stitched up. I was dead tired and went to sleep in A&E under her bed. Eventually, when all was settled, I crept away to go home. I got as far as the door before a nurse told me I could not go home because my back was still bleeding; my sweater was soaked with Mary's blood. It was a different day out at the seaside.

Parkinson's and falls are a way of life. We now have a plethora of devices leading to a rollator, but the falls still continue.

When a serious fall happens, inevitably it's 999 and the ambulance service that come to the rescue, but sadly—as a result of the deterioration of the NHS, the pandemic and strikes—confidence has gone. After another fall, Mary was taken to hospital. She lay on a trolley, without medical attention, for ten hours. I took her home without treatment being given, although her face and head were badly bruised.

However, life goes on and Mary is very determined to stay upright. She has continued with tai chi and instructions from her iPad, although we know any improvement is bound to be transitory. If she has had a persistent problem, over the years, it has been me. She cannot articulate with clarity and my deafness has not improved, so communication has to be well planned. The ten-year age gap between us has become a big problem. Almost without a pause I have had one problem after another and that has affected her life too. One thing is for sure: we have helped each other. If we had remained alone, life would have become very difficult for both of us.

My PSA was increasing. Digital tests and scans were inconclusive, as was a biopsy through my backside and bowel; unfortunately, infections followed. These tests continued from 2013 to 2017. Then I was given a general anaesthetic and forty-seven very long needles were stuck into the area under my testicles and into the front of the prostate. Cancer was found and a few needles had evidence of advanced cancer. I decided, at the age of seventy-nine, to live with the cancer and I was advised to become concerned if I lived long enough for the PSA to rise to 40, or if the rate of increase was 50% during a single year. I was to watch and wait. The final biopsy caused a setback in my health; I bled and looked bruised around my private parts for somewhile. Nevertheless, I became fit again. I even did some windsurfing and played golf regularly. Then came the accident.

Every Monday, whatever the weather, I joined a group of friends to play golf at Crane Valley, near Verwood. One autumnal Monday, after there had been rain, heavy rain, the ground was very muddy underfoot. Most players were finding conditions exceedingly difficult. When we arrived at the par 3 sixth hole there was a queue at the tee, which was elevated with a steep slope and a set of steps. The time was filled in with some banter from me at the bottom of the slope and the waiting group at the tee. Then came one of the consequences of my deafness. In order to hear a rude remark aimed at me, I heaved myself up the slope then turned round to go back to my position in the queue. As I turned round, my right foot shot away and I headed down the slope on my backside. The fall was gentle and normally we would have all laughed it off. There probably were some amused chuckles, but my left leg was on a journey of its own.

When the rest of my body passed it, there was a loud cracking noise that reverberated through my body. The rest of the golfers must have heard the sound because they went quiet and the silence was only broken by some extreme expletives from me, enveloped in pain. When I reached the bottom of the slope I attempted to stand. The pain was excruciating, and the expletives were repeated at such volume they could be heard on the fifth and seventh holes. I collapsed back into a heap. The ligaments in my quads had been totally torn away from my kneecap. My left leg was now misfunctioning in two separate parts.

My golfing partners and the club professional did a marvellous job to get me to the clubhouse, and a paramedic and ambulance were quick to arrive. Morphine was gratefully received. My family was informed and that was the start of tea and sympathy. From A&E I was taken to X-ray and from there I was soon under another general anaesthetic and in the operating theatre. The ligaments were collected together with strapping and that was connected by another strap to a pin in my kneecap. The bottom and top of my leg were reconnected, and I continued my journey to become Bionic Man.

As ever, that was not the end but the start of problems. Tina came to the rescue by helping Mary to gather clothes and suchlike that were easy to put over stiff and unfriendly limbs. Yet again I had to start a recovery period that involved crutches, sticks, stretching and exercises. I told my doctor I was not going to walk with a stick for the rest of my life; I would return to windsurfing and golf.

"Terry, I quite understand. When they put you in a box, there will be no stick."

Well, windsurfing declined but I continued to play golf and I told myself to hold my head up high and walk with a straight back. I know the doctor was telling me something about my bloody-mindedness; I am not that insensitive. After that incident, windsurfing became a thing of the past and I seldom ventured on to a golf course, but I needed to keep fit to look after Mary. I walked, stretched and eventually walked without a limp. If I hadn't moved for an hour or so, I would go for a walk and drink coffee. In two years, my Fitbit recorded 5,000 kilometres and I spent a small fortune on coffee. It was worth the effort! My blood pressure reduced, and my BMI came close to perfection. Despite the problems of the pandemic and an early bout of Covid and sepsis, I survived.

When I eventually saw my doctor, he said, in some amazement, "Terry, you're still alive."

At eighty-four years old, that was good news.

Chapter Twenty-Six
The Pandemic

The year 2020 was going to be difficult for everybody—right across the world. It all started around January or February with some news that there was another SARS-type virus in China transmitted by eating bats or snakes and suchlike. Or maybe it was even man-made? But it was in China and China was a long way away. It was just passing news.

However, the spread of the virus and its effects were soon to dominate all that we did and thought.

In February things came closer to home. There was the news of a new coronavirus spreading under the name of COVID-19. The outbreak was spreading across China and people were dying. The fear that it would spread internationally became a reality, especially as so many Chinese students were returning to British universities. Almost immediately, there were outbreaks at French and Italian ski resorts. The UK government went into a dither, even though travel through our airports was widely recognised to be a growing problem. At this time, Mary's family was heading south to visit us and Thomas's journey became convoluted. He visited Edinburgh, Manchester and Southampton airports. I was concerned.

However, the visit went well, and the family went back to Edinburgh. Then we learnt they had gone down with a virus, which was diagnosed as an adenovirus. They were quite ill and went back and forth to hospital. I have often wondered, *Was it an adenovirus?* There was no testing at this stage.

Mary and I had booked a weekend away at Falmouth in February, and an impending pandemic was acknowledged, but no particular action had been announced. It was a great weekend and our first lengthy venture in an electric car. We took a break at Exeter and stopped for lunch and an EV charge at a nice farm shop. We enjoyed the weekend walking around the city and visiting the Maritime Museum. By now Coronavirus was dominating the news and I was conscious of a cruise ship, with American passengers, and Chinese students in the coffee shops. But still no word from the Government about what the country should do.

A couple of weeks after we returned from Falmouth, Covid was becoming quite serious and then in mid-March it happened.

First came a slight sore throat, then a bit of a headache, and one evening I felt very cold; so cold, in fact, that I went to bed to get warm. I *did* get nice and warm and then I became hot. This was followed by sweats and the bed was soaked. The coughing started and would not stop. I coughed so much my chest and arms ached. I staggered through the next day. Then, when I moved away from Mary to get some tea, I collapsed to the ground and my heart rate shot up to 170 beats per minute. At my age then, my maximum heart rate should have been no more than 140. My temperature was 38° Celsius. I rang 111 but became impatient and gave up. The news was now full of the virus and its implications.

A few days later, after I had already put myself in isolation, the country followed. I tried to get a test, as tests were starting up at Southampton, but I had to give up. I decided, come what may, I would look after myself. Mary had a slight cough, which did not get worse, and I was grateful for that. My coughing stopped after about five days and I felt better, but this was followed by over eight months of other problems. Although I was never tested, I believe I was suffering from what became known as "long Covid".

The first problem was being tired, accompanied by foggy spells which stayed for a long while. Then came sciatica. Talking to the surgery about it became difficult. However, I eventually received some painkillers, which I took although they had side effects. My back got better and "Lockdown 1" ended. I tried to play golf, but the sciatica returned with a vengeance. I managed to get an X-ray and was told my back was old, like the rest of my body. Then I went to a physio who told me it was not necessarily my old spine that was the problem but groups of muscles around my spine and diaphragm. He said I needed to learn to breathe again. I later learned that this difficulty in breathing was an aspect of long Covid. I stretched to work off the problem and went to the gym, but I had to be careful because my cardio belt was telling me my heart was unstable and would "run away" if I exercised even gently. At night, breathing produced aches in my chest, which decreased when I was standing. Sleeping produced nightmares and then I developed insomnia. The doctor said I was under tension. Well, he was right about that!

Every day I stretched, walked and went to the gym—when it was open. I wrote to my doctor describing the symptoms and saying I thought I had Covid and long Covid. He replied via the receptionist: "Noted."

I told my family I had Covid, but it was such early days they were sceptical. Were they just the meanderings of an old man? However, we were to learn later that the majority of deaths were amongst people of my age suffering at home. My physical fitness, correct BMI and vitamin D3 supplement may have saved me. March to September was a truly difficult period when I fought in isolation except for Mary's support.

To add to my woes, in September I had a blood test to check on my prostate cancer. The readings had reached a critical PSA of nearly 40 and I spoke to my doctor. Covid was now dominating the NHS. I felt things were difficult, and it didn't help that a *Times Insight* exposé had revealed that eighty year olds were being given a secret triage rating that suggested they should be kept away from hospitals. I cheekily asked what my rating was and there was deafening silence. I took the silence as agreement that the over-eighties had been rated and put into a separate box.

I got over the embarrassing talk with my doctor and decided to write directly to the hospital consultant. He told me my cancer had most likely spread from the prostate and then spoke with great candour and consideration, for now it was a toss of the die as to whether I died of a heart attack, a stroke or the ravages of cancer. He kept talking of his dilemma and, in retrospect, I realised I had gone over the head of my GP; the consultant now had to find a solution that kept me clear of hospital.

I elected to fight cancer. I was to be given initial medication (an LHRH injection), which would take away any drive and make me tired. I was liable to lose muscle mass and bone density. The most serious effect, however, was that I was going to be chemically castrated. It seemed that LHRH was not appropriate, and I was prescribed bicalutamide daily, which was given with tamoxifen on the assumption that the cancer had spread and there was a danger of breast cancer. The side effects were life-changing and were probably exacerbated by long Covid; they made caring for, and living with, Mary exceedingly difficult. I was, however, kept away from hospital. The treatment was administered by prescription from the local surgery.

In the midst of my fight, came the euphoria of Covid vaccination. The Government had, sensibly, contracted to buy enough vaccines to cover the population over eighteen years of age. The process started with the vulnerable and the over-eighties, who started to receive doses in December 2020. I received my first dose of the Pfizer vaccine on 20th December and the one-and-only, long-promised LHRH prostate injection on Christmas Eve, prior to starting the course of bicalutamide. I felt unwell for a while, but I was looking forward to having more freedom to do household tasks after I had the booster jab on 10th January. I had calculated that Mary would get her first Covid injection sometime in February. Things were looking good, especially when it seemed possible that I might "buy some time" when I was to be tested for PSA in March 2021. Expectations were high, and morale increased.

I was later to discover something about bicalutamide. It was an old drug for treating prostate cancer that had spread, but that was only an assumption in my case. Later, I paid for scans that revealed the cancer was confined to my prostate. Age and circumstances had made getting tests unnecessarily difficult.

It had been convenient for the hospital to keep me away, on the reckoning I would die out of sight and out of mind during the time of the pandemic and incredible chaos in the NHS. I eventually made a personal decision and stopped taking bicalutamide and tamoxifen and asked for the situation to be reviewed.

Over the two years that I had been fighting the side effects, I routinely continued stretching, using weights and walking. I kept my weight down and ate a balanced diet. I had been abandoned by the NHS, but I would fight alone. I literally walked thousands of kilometres to control my weight and blood pressure, but the price I paid was having to endure periods of extreme fatigue caused by medical side effects and old age.

There is a Jewish expression: "Man plans, and God laughs."

So it was that expectations started to fade. The administration of Pfizer jabs had been regulated. Pfizer recommended that vaccinations should be three weeks apart, but the Government decided that the time before the second injection should be extended to up to twelve weeks so the first dose could be spread more widely. Pfizer had declared that the first dose would provide 52% immunity over a wait of three weeks. A government announcement suggested that immunity was misunderstood, and it could be as high as 90%. It was a gamble. I wrote to the BBC questioning such an arbitrary decision and suggesting it could cause chaos. The BBC put me on national news. Consequently, that put me in contact with friends from the past. (We subsequently learned that the medical profession was also not convinced of the validity of extending the gap between vaccinations.)

It seemed strange to me that the Government did not want to test their decision. After all, it could turn out to be valid and the data collection would have been reassuring.

Israel had been encouraged to vaccinate early with a contractual trial for Pfizer and there had been suggestions that the first dose had not been 52% efficient but could give as low as 30% immunity. As time passed, this proved to be wrong, and the vaccinations were shown to be much more effective than first thought. A problem arose with the AstraZeneca vaccine and a few people died of blood clots on the brain. Even though the vaccine was very successful, confidence was lost for a while.

I continued to suffer during 2021 with two more bouts of sciatica, the side effects of cancer treatment, extreme lethargy, random aches and pains, a UTI and sepsis. I could not tell what was caused by long Covid and what was due to prostate treatment, but the good news was that my PSA fell from 40 to 0.5. However, during this period I got angry with the off-handedness of my surgery and Primary Care, and

I wrote to the Minister of Health, Matt Hancock (of *I'm a Celebrity Get Me Out of Here*), and the Director of Primary Care and told them what I thought about their triaging and organisation. While I proved my point, my outrage did not go down well, especially with my local surgery. The NHS and Primary Care seemed to be breaking apart.[24]

I slowly realised that ageism had become part of our culture and had been endorsed by our prime minister during the pandemic. What a fool he was, but the electorate had voted for him, and he conned those who had believed in him. He had declared that many over-eighties had died during the pandemic, but that was the way life (death) was, and we all owed the younger generation for their tolerance. I think he had future Conservative voting strength in mind because many of the aged would be dead by the next election. His concern about his own inflated status became very apparent and dominated over sensible decision-making during the months that followed. His stupidity was to destroy him as PM and as an MP, and the Conservative Party seemed to join the chaos of the NHS, or was it the other way round?[25]

While Mary was away in Edinburgh during this difficult period, I started to feel very ill. I tried to get

---

[24] I was right; the linkage between Primary Care and the hospitals remains in a bad way.

[25] My comments were written before he was charged for breaking the law by flouting Covid rules, and he resigned as an MP.

help from my GP and failed yet again. The doctor was late for our telephone appointment. He, also, was stressed and was intolerant of my poor hearing and my confused state. He put the phone down and left me in the lurch. I went to bed and slept. When I woke in the night, I thought I was going to pass out. I rang 111 and an ambulance came. The following hours were but a blur. I had realised how difficult things could become for an old person alone at home with a developing illness.

When I left hospital, the doctor said I had had a UTI, but my departure document recorded sepsis as well; I gather the two may be linked. I had developed a fever, evacuated everything out of my body, lost half a stone and then slowly recovered due to the excellent skills of the doctors and nurses in the hospital.

Despite my stress there was an incident that amused me. As I lay half asleep in my bed on the morning following the initial crisis and a traumatic night, I felt a gentle kiss on my cheek. I awoke to find an old lady taking pity on me. I was alive and grateful for her kindness.

I do not think I would have survived had I not rung 111. Sepsis is a serious condition. Permission was given for me to be taken home by Chris and Tina, to start another recovery as best I could.

Mary returned from Edinburgh. I felt better. I

helped in the garden during the following weeks, then really hurt my back and left leg through another form of sciatica. I entered yet another three-month recovery period before walking again. My left leg, with damaged ligaments, was a real problem. I was determined to walk again and, little by little, my walking got better. I was eventually walking over thirty miles a week, but between bouts of tiredness. During this period, the truth about the NHS and seven million people on the waiting lists emphasised that Mary and I, like so many others, were in for a lonely fight in our terminal years.

It was unsurprising that mental health was given a great deal of publicity on the internet during the bad times of the pandemic. The loss of NHS capability has featured too often in the media, to the point it has grown large in people's minds. My scribblings have shown that when things get bad it is easier now, more than in the past, to think about the possibility of suicide. Strangely, during the last two years I have looked into the abyss and each time I have decided to fight, as in the case recorded in the prologue to my book about middle life. Above all is the thought that I cannot abandon Mary.

I have been outraged by members of the community and Government who do selfish and stupid things, especially in this difficult period and I have asked myself: *Should I be more tolerant for they can-*

not help it? They are just being human.[26] With this thought in my mind, I took counselling.

I did not know that a year later there would be something akin to a general strike. Initially, I had some sympathy for the strikers but it slowly vaporised, especially for the junior doctors who were members of the BMA. I was to witness another failure of A&E for Mary, much as it had been for Trish. Mary had fallen, hit her head again and been taken to hospital. She waited in A&E for eight hours without food and water, and had not been seen by a doctor. She became distraught and I brought her home when I found she was walking unaided looking for a toilet. Later in the day I took her back to get a scan and see a doctor. It was the first day of the junior doctors' strike. Any sympathy I might have had turned to anger. I wrote long comments in *The Times* about greed and the lack of thought for the disadvantaged part of society.

Despite my successful fight for survival, I felt there was nothing to lose by talking about the pressure I was under. I had two long sessions with a counsellor and the second session was particularly searching. She said I was obviously a passionate man and had squeezed a great deal of activity into my life; she wanted to know how I thought I had affected

---

26 I became particularly annoyed with senior NHS doctors striking for more money when others in society were having a desperate struggle.

other people's lives. There was obviously my large family and my two wives, and I had tried to spread my time and energy across many locations and tasks. Many times, I had felt it was all beyond my capability and I felt guilt for what had been imposed on my family. I told her I hadn't given much thought to how I had affected colleagues and people who had worked for me, but over the last few years several people who had been associated with me fifty to sixty years ago had sought me out to thank me for being me and for things I had said and done; I had affected their lives and careers positively. At the time it had greatly surprised me and, as I recalled these events, I had to pull back tears of embarrassment. It had given me joy to learn that I had affected lives in the very best of ways.

Then came the counsellor's advice. I will try to encapsulate it: "You are very self-critical, but you have done so much. Just be proud of that, for you have obviously affected people in a good way. You can do little more now, but my advice is to be more selfish and take more care of yourself."

As I stood up at the end of the meeting, I was really shaken by her last comment: "My father was your age. He had a big heart and I miss him. He died of the effects of Covid and long Covid a few weeks ago."

Like most people, the counsellor had her problems.

She had been so brave to carry out that interview and the full meaning of her advice hit home very hard in the year to follow.

Chapter Twenty-Seven
The World Is Broken, the UK Is Broken, the NHS Is Broken; We Fight On

When celebrities write their memoirs they are mostly limited to a series of similar events and a limited period of time. I have tried to cover my lifetime in two books. I am beginning to realise, regardless of the quality of the writing, that I have climbed a mountain, and I am almost at the top looking down.

In previous paragraphs I wrote about the Covid pandemic. It affected me badly, like so many others in my age group. We have had pandemics before and coped, but along came 2022. I was to learn that my kidneys were starting to fail and, more importantly, we became swamped with worldwide problems that have enveloped all of us. Over the top of everything lie the problems associated with climate change. Fine words are mouthed but action is thin. Brexit took the UK away from the EU and, when the pandemic arrived, the Tory Party became split and lost control. Then followed the Russians' invasion of Ukraine which affected the worldwide distribution of energy and food. Russia and China started to show signs of instability and that instability spread across the world to the US, the Sudan, Iran, other parts of the Middle East, and even France and the old Soviet Union countries in Eastern Europe. And along came the devastating conflict between Hamas and Israel!

There has also been the return of inflation, which affected the UK most of all, partly because of Brexit. It was the start of an on-off recession (my analysis, not that of the Bank of England who kept saying we were close). The big problem had been the printing of money, called, euphemistically, quantitative easing.

At the beginning of this millennium there were a lot of prophecies about what might, or might not, happen around the year 2000. There have been the Ages of the Hunter-Gatherer, Agriculture, and Industrialisation. We have now entered the Age of Information and Artificial Intelligence. No one took much notice at first, but there is a new form of chaos. There is also a rottenness at the very top of business and even amongst the politicians. The same sort of issue had already appeared with the fall of Communism and the generation of the oligarchs. Those who got to grips with the change became the super-rich and societies split even more than in the past. I like the quote of Danny Hillis, who wrote about this subject at the turn of the millennium:[27]

> *"It feels like something big is about to happen. Graphs show us the yearly growth of populations, atmospheric concentration of carbon dioxide, net addresses, and Mbytes per dollar. They all soar up to an asymptote just beyond the turn of the century: the Singularity. The end of all we know. The beginning of something we may never understand."*

It is more than twenty-three years since we entered the new millennium, but I still warm to the quote. It seems so very true. Now there is even talk that artificial intelligence may destroy humanity. This is the setting for the last years of my life and with the "Fourth Age", as described, I write on about my existence in its cauldron while I swirl, inevitably, to infinity.

If I stand back and look at our situation, my luck—while it still prevails—is getting thin. The clouds are there, but the shadow is hard to discern. Mary has coped with Parkinson's amazingly over a period of twenty-five years and she fights to keep fit so she can see her grandsons, but the fight is coming to an end and the winters of 2022 and 2023 were difficult in so many ways. I am registered to care for her, but I

---

[27] Danny Hillis is an inventor, scientist, author and engineer. He pioneered the concept of building highly parallel computers. His knowledge, patents and achievements are huge. I think he should add "philosopher" to his métiers.

am not sure who is going to care for whom. In health terms, people of our age are being triaged away from a national health system that is falling apart. There is a need for private investment in health if we are to defeat waiting times.

Brexit caused difficulties, but the Tory government was already in disarray, with chaos caused by the almost annual change of prime ministers. The last thing the Tories will ever want to do is admit their mistakes. Frankly, they got into the habit of lying to cover bad decisions and misdeeds. It was bad enough that they had to recognise the stupidity of taking the wrong road at a time of severe inflation and a looming recession, but their excuse was always the tremendous job they said they had done during the pandemic. However, I am not so sure of their claimed success; a long-drawn-out investigation of the government's actions may eventually discover the truth. The scientists did a great job producing vaccines that may even become a way forward in treating cancers, but some MPs put their snouts in the trough and made a fortune. They also dallied and partied while the population was in lockdown. While some politicians tried to do their best, their work was stained by others who behaved very badly.

Then came Putin's attack on the Ukraine and it arrived bringing increasing inflation in the UK and across the world. Along came a hard winter and an energy crisis. For a couple of years, I have been pessimistic about inflation. It was not that I was gifted with prescience; it was just that things had the same smell as in the 1970s. I said as much to a banker friend and another friend who was a committed Tory, and they told me not to be so stupid. It was a global glitch and would be over quite quickly. Then came the Russian invasion and these friends of mine said it would be over in a week. In fact, there was a general feeling in the media that Russia was so strong that the Ukraine would be decimated. I remembered my training during the Cold War and the problems of attack on an embedded defence of a homeland, especially one that was over great distances. I said the Ukrainians would dig in and it would go on for a much longer time than was generally thought. Of course, I did not know that the West would support Ukraine, or that Putin would cut off energy supplies to Europe or that he would blitz or drown Ukrainian civilians when a military battle had not gone his way. But it was easy to forecast that Putin had constructed a situation that was not too far from that of Hitler and Stalin.

At one stage I was rude in *The Times* about his brain and stature and said any intelligent person could see his false flag flying ahead of his "special operation" and invasion threat. Within three hours I had a call from Moscow. When I answered with my name the phone was put down. I traced the call but could not get a reply.[28] There has been but a pause in the Cold War and yet again, as with the demise of the Soviet Union, Russia is entering a period that could possibly bring a civil war and even nuclear threats. The wheel, as ever, turns again, but I am not sure I will have time left to see much of an improvement.

---

28 The telephone call was two weeks before the "Special Operation". Perhaps the call was understandable. My name must be somewhere on KGB records. It would have been documented that I had been a squadron commander and an intelligence officer to an admiral. They probably also knew my age and that would have been the end of any investigation.

Epilogue
Accepting the Inevitable

My memoirs have covered eighty-five years and two volumes. Readers will have to judge my book. I think it has been an achievement, but now it is time for me to stop, for the end is in sight. My writings have little value in the world at large, but the big value has been that, like a computer system, I have a cloud and I can access it as a back-up to my memory. My memory would surely have faded much more quickly without my writing.

My original intention was to write for my grandchildren because I knew little or nothing about *my* grandparents and I did not want history to repeat itself. My family has made little or no comment, but one of my friends commented, "Terry, your writing is brutally honest." I take that as a positive remark. After all, there is little point in bending the truth. I know some in my family will see things differently from me because, although we are related, we have trodden different paths.

The histories in my two books are very different and display the big difference between youthful energy and the grind of old age. There has always been the fight for survival but in this later life of "fading luck", it is more about the maintenance of health, very different from the risk-taking in early life.

My story is unique, but I am sure most families have a story to tell. Dare they tell it?

Abbreviations Used

AMRAAM	advanced medium-range air-to-air missile
ASRAAM	advanced short-range air-to-air missile
A&E	accident and emergency department
BAE	British Aeronautical Engineering
BFA	British Funboard Association
BMI	body mass index
BVR	beyond visual range
B&B	bed and breakfast
CCF	Combined Cadet Force/Central Control Function
CGI	computer-generated imagery
CQC	Care Quality Commission
CSF	Compagnie Générale de Télégraphie Sans Fil (General Wireless Telegraphy Company)
DEW	directed energy weapons
ECG	electrocardiogram
FIRS	flight information regions
IBM	International Business Machines (a multinational technology company)
ITP	invitation to participate

LHRH	luteinising hormone-releasing hormone (a hormone that stimulates the production of the hormones that start puberty)
MAD	mutual assured destruction
MOD	Ministry of Defence
NATS	National Air Traffic System
N^{2}EMP	non-nuclear electromagnetic pulse
OA	operational assessment
OAP	old age pensioner
PCT	primary care trust
P.E.	physical education
PFI	private finance initiative
PSA	prostate-specific antigen. The PSA test is a blood test to help detect prostate cancer.
Radman	Research and Development Management Limited
RAF	Royal Air Force
RN	Royal Navy
RYA	Royal Yachting Association
SDI	Strategic Defense Initiative
UKBSA	United Kingdom Board Sailing Association
USAF	United States Air Force
UTI	urinary tract infection
WFH	working from home

Glossary

dolmen	a megalithic tomb with a large flat stone laid on upright ones
dyskinesia	a movement disorder that often appears as uncontrolled shakes, tics or tremors
gybe	to change course by swinging the sail across the following wind

Additional Information

BIC	a French manufacturing corporation that produces pens, razors and other disposable products, as well as water sports products
Thomson-CSF	a French company that specialises in the development and manufacture of electronics with a heavy focus upon the aerospace and defence sectors of the market

Printed in Great Britain
by Amazon